WITHDRAWN

Human Rights and Public Health in the AIDS Pandemic

Human Rights and Public Health in the AIDS Pandemic

LAWRENCE O. GOSTIN, J.D., LL.D. (HON.)
Professor of Law, Georgetown University Law Center
Co-Director, Georgetown/Johns Hopkins University Program
on Law and Public Health

ZITA LAZZARINI, J.D., M.P.H.
Lecturer, Harvard School of Public Health

New York   Oxford
OXFORD UNIVERSITY PRESS
1997

Oxford University Press

Oxford New York
Athens Auckland Bangkok Bogota
Bombay Buenos Aires Calcutta Cape Town
Dar es Salaam Delhi Florence Hong Kong Istanbul
Karachi Kuala Lumpur Madras Madrid
Melbourne Mexico City Nairobi Paris
Singapore Taipei Tokyo Toronto

and associated companies in
Berlin Ibadan

Library of Congress Cataloging-in-Publication Data
Gostin, Larry O. (Larry Ogalthorpe)
Human rights and public health in the AIDS pandemic /
Lawrence O. Gostin, Zita Lazzarini.
p. cm. Includes bibliographical references and index.
ISBN 0-19-511442-6
1. AIDS (Disease)—Patients—Legal status, laws, etc.
2. Public health laws.
3. Human rights. 4. Public health—Government policy.
I. Lazzarini, Zita.
II. Title.
K3575.A43G67 1997 349.73'08'80814—dc20 [347.300880814] 96-33501

9 8 7 6 5 4 3 2 1

Printed in the United States of America
on acid-free paper

For

Jean, Bryn, and Kieran
(L.O.G.)

Gary, Ariel, Lucca, and Salem
(Z.L.)

Foreword

The Universal Declaration of Human Rights begins with a recognition of the inherent dignity and the equal and inalienable rights of all people. This is also where the fundamental relationship between human rights, health, and non-discrimination is embedded, giving rise to a highly topical human rights issue, namely that of human rights of people living with HIV/AIDS. The relationship between human rights and HIV/AIDS is complex: the protection of human rights is necessary to reduce vulnerability to HIV infection and to eliminate all forms of discrimination practised against those living with HIV/ AIDS, their families, and friends.

It is not necessary to recount the numerous charters and declarations on HIV/AIDS and human rights to understand human rights in the context of HIV/AIDS. All persons are born free and equal in dignity and rights. Everyone, including persons seeking to avoid HIV infection, as well as persons living with HIV/AIDS, is entitled to all the rights and freedoms set forth in the international human rights instruments without discrimination, such as the rights to life, liberty, security of person, privacy, health, education, work, social security, and to marry and found a family. Yet, violations of human rights in the context of HIV/AIDS are a reality to be found in every corner of the globe.

Public health should not be used by states as a justification for coercive powers against persons living with HIV/AIDS. Measures such as the loss of liberty and discriminatory practices in employment, housing, education, insurance and travel continue to affect people living with HIV/AIDS in many countries. Yet, coercive and discriminatory powers do not necessarily promote public health. Coercion and discrimination, by driving people away from prevention and treatment services, can fuel the HIV/AIDS pandemic. One clear message needs to be sent: respect for human rights and advancement of the public health are not in conflict, but in harmony. People cannot fully enjoy and exercise their human rights if they are not healthy, and people cannot remain healthy if they are deprived of their rights.

There exists, therefore, an obligation by states to provide populations, within the limits of their resources, with prevention services, including clear and targeted health information necessary to reduce their risk of contracting HIV infection. It is critically important that individuals and groups be granted access to information necessary to make informed choices about their health as well as the means to protect themselves, in a manner consistent with universally recognized human rights standards yet reconciled within different cultures and religions.

Some groups in society suffering from discrimination in the enjoyment of their fundamental rights and freedoms, such as women and children, are frequently at disproportionally higher risk of HIV/AIDS infection. Substantial efforts are needed by governments and society to protect the rights of such vulnerable groups at the international, national, and local levels. Effective and action-oriented measures to improve their disadvantaged legal, social, and economic status would not only assure the protection of their human rights and fundamental freedoms, but would also lower the risk of HIV infection.

The social and legal status of women in many societies illustrates the connectedness of HIV/AIDS and human rights. Laws, traditions, customs, and practices in some cultures and religions promote the subordinate status and exploitation of women in marriages and relationships, thereby directly increasing women's and their children's vulnerability to HIV infection. The protection of human rights of children is indispensable to avoid their infection or for them to be able to cope when confronted with HIV/AIDS. To guarantee freedom from sexual exploitation and trafficking is even more critical in view of the HIV/AIDS pandemic.

Professor Gostin and Ms. Lazzarini develop with clarity and rigor the fundamental relationships between health and human rights. Their book, and its message of respect for human rights and the promotion of health, demands attention both within the human rights community and the public health community.

As Professor Gostin and Ms. Lazzarini explain in their text, for far too long public health professionals have regarded human rights as peripheral to their interests, failing to see how critical human rights are to achieving improved health for the population. Human rights groups have yet to find the most effective way to integrate health-related, and in particular HIV/AIDS, concerns in their mandates. Our purpose in jointly writing this foreword is to dispel these myths and overcome prevailing apathies. We ask our respective communities to see the synergy between public health and human rights and to embrace both in their important work. The journey begins with a recognition of the inherent dignity and equal rights of all people and an understanding that the protection of human health is indispensable for the protection of the human rights and fundamental freedoms of everyone.

Peter Piot
Executive Director, Joint United Nations Programme on HIV/AIDS
José Ayala-Lasso
United Nations High Commissioner for Human Rights

Acknowledgments

We owe a great intellectual debt to many organizations and individuals who have worked tirelessly on the relationships between health and human rights. The Joint United Nations Programme on HIV/AIDS (UNAIDS)—cosponsored by the United Nations International Children's Educational Fund (UNICEF), the United Nations Development Programme (UNDP), the United Nations Fund for Population Activity (UNFPA), the United Nations Educational, Scientific and Cultural Organization (UNESCO), the World Health Organization (WHO), and the World Bank—was instrumental in facilitating this book. The approach of UNAIDS, energetically led by Peter Piot, is that the HIV/AIDS pandemic affects not only public health, but also the economy, educational and resource capabilities, development gains, and human rights within countries. Susan Timberlake, human rights adviser for UNAIDS, has been indispensable not only in relation to this book but in her leadership in bridging the human rights and HIV/AIDS communities.

The original idea for this book arose when one of us (L.O.G.) led the staff at the World Health Organization Global Programme on AIDS (GPA) in an in-house reflection on human rights during the summer of 1991 in Geneva at the invitation of Michael Merson and Dorothy Blake. Several legal and human rights officers for GPA, including Katarina Tomasevski, Lane Porter, and Kelvin Widdows, provided valuable comments and guidance throughout the process. The rigorous work of Sev Fluss, then Chief of Health Legislation and now human rights coordinator at WHO, has been invaluable. Dr. Zbigniew Bankowski, Director of the Council of International Organizations of Medical Sciences (CIOMS), contributed richly to our thinking about the research questions explored in this book.

The fundamental connections between health and human rights, and generally between AIDS and human rights, have been the subject of ongoing interest for a wonderful group of friends and colleagues at the Harvard School of Public Health's François-Xavier Bagnoud Center on Health and Human Rights. Group discussions have informed our research and teaching, as well as our personal concern and dedication to international human rights. Jonathan Mann, François-Xavier Bagnoud Professor of Health and Human Rights, has been an inspirational colleague in exploring the relationship between public health and human rights. He was particularly instrumental in development of the human rights impact assessment and jointly authored the first publication of its principles (Gostin, Mann, 1994). Sophia Gruskin also richly participated in our discussions of the human rights impact assessment.

We are also grateful to our colleagues in the Georgetown /Johns Hopkins University Program on Law and Public Health. Those deserving of special mention are Dean Judith Areen, who provided a Dean's Scholarship Award for this research; professors Gregg Bloche and Carlos Vazquez, who cotaught a workshop at Georgetown University Law Center with one of us (L.O.G.) on human rights; and Ruth Faden and Stephen Teret in the Program on Law, Ethics, and Health at the Johns Hopkins University School of Hygiene and Public Health.

We also are grateful to our students at Harvard Law School, Harvard School of Public Health, Georgetown University Law Center, and the Johns Hopkins School of Hygiene and Public Health for their enthusiasm and intellectual rigor in health and human rights courses. We hope to see the curricula of many Schools of Public Health, Medicine, Nursing, and Law incorporate concepts of health and human rights.

A number of dedicated professionals in public health, medicine, and jurisprudence assisted in the creation of this book. Elizabeth H. Abi-Mershed, staff attorney, Inter-American Commission on Human Rights, deserves special recognition for her conceptualization of the human rights framework discussed early in the book. The following individuals have also been indispensable to the completion of this book, and their contribution is deeply appreciated: Susan Stayn, then a human rights intern at Columbia University School of Law; Kathleen Flaherty, then an editor of the *Harvard Human Rights Law Journal*; and Kathleen Maguire, currently with Georgetown–Johns Hopkins University Program on Law and Public Health. Susan Yeon and Madeline Stein, Harvard Law School; Tamyra Comeaux, Harvard AIDS Institute and Morehouse School of Medicine; and Deirdre Kamber, Hofstra University Law School, also contributed their talents and energies. Warm thanks also go to Professor Ronald Bayer, Columbia University School of Public Health, for thoughtful comments on the manuscript.

Rich and important work on AIDS and human rights enlightened and inspired our thinking. Among many distinctive contributions by individuals and organizations are those of Michael Kirby (High Court of Australia), Julia Hausermann (Rights and Humanity), Elizabeth Reid (United Nations Development Programme), Renee Sabatier (formerly at the Panos Institute), Helen Watchirs (Attorney General's Department, Australia), the late Paul Sieghart (the British Medical Association), and Luis Varela Quiros (United Nations, Special Rapporteur). The collective thinking and action of these and many other highly valued colleagues and advocates will, we hope, bring greater appreciation of the fundamental importance of human rights in AIDS and public health.

Finally, and most important, we want to dedicate this book to our families, the realm in which health and human respect find truest expression.

Washington, D.C.   L. O. G.
Boston, Massachusetts   Z. L.
August 1996

Contents

Introduction

The AIDS pandemic presents a major challenge to public health and human rights. The burden of HIV/AIDS is borne disproportionately by people and communities already suffering from poverty, hunger, homelessness, inadequate health care, discrimination, and stigmatization. The pandemic has caused enormous suffering throughout the world. The Joint United Nations Programme on HIV/AIDS reports that as of June 1996, nearly 1.3 million people have AIDS, a twenty-five percent increase over a year earlier (United Nations [UNAIDS], 1996c). UNAIDS estimates that twenty-one million adults are currently infected with HIV, and that number is projected to climb to forty million individuals by the year 2000. By then, nine of ten HIV-infected individuals will live in developing countries and rates of new infection in parts of Asia and Latin America likely will match or exceed present rates in Africa. Tragically, AIDS will become a leading cause of death in children, with more than ten million infected by the end of the decade (United Nations [UNAIDS], 1996b; World Health Organization, 1993, 1992b).

From a public health perspective, HIV/AIDS is fundamentally connected with the pandemics of drug abuse (Porter, Gostin, 1992; Normand, Vlahov, et al., 1995), sexually transmitted diseases (Laga, Nzila, et al., 1991), and tuberculosis (DeCock, Soro, et al., 1992). These global health problems will profoundly influence the future epidemiology of HIV/AIDS and will intensify the challenge of prevention as well as the treatment and care of persons living with HIV/AIDS.

Like other blood-borne diseases, HIV/AIDS is transmitted primarily in three ways: through sexual intercourse; through exposure to contaminated drug injection or medical equipment; and from mother-to-child transmission during pregnancy, birth, or breast-feeding. There is no evidence that people are at risk of infection from casual or prolonged contact with someone living with HIV/AIDS. The actual nature of the risk of infection and the *non-communicability* of HIV/AIDS under most circumstances have profound implications for policymakers in designing HIV/AIDS prevention programs.

The burden of the AIDS pandemic extends well beyond public health. HIV/AIDS poses incalculable human, social, cultural, and economic costs. The effects pervade the industrial, agricultural, and health care sectors and permeate society, affecting individuals, families, and communities (Hanson, 1992). HIV/AIDS primarily affects younger and middle-aged people. The death of a parent or wage earner often leaves dependents (both young and old) poor, malnourished, and homeless (Commonwealth Secretariat, 1990).

On the deepest human level, it is hardly possible to convey the degree of human suffering unleashed in a community ravaged by HIV/AIDS. Countless children grow up without parents and end up roaming through villages or living on the street. People see their loved ones, family members, and friends sapped of health and vitality, and soon, of life itself. In some parts of the world, the disease breaks up families and inflicts such social and economic harm that it threatens the destruction of communities altogether.

There are several disciplinary approaches that could usefully illuminate the social, legal, and ethical aspects of HIV/AIDS. One method of examination used by scholars focuses on the philosophic or ethical framework of autonomy, beneficence, and distributive justice (Bayer, 1991; Daniels, 1985, 1995). While this text borrows from this ethical discourse, its principal method of examination is the body of international law codified in the International Bill of Human Rights.

All persons are born with and possess throughout their lives a set of entitlements which the international community terms human rights. Human rights embody a set of fundamental claims to life, liberty, and equality of opportunity that cannot be taken away by the government, persons, or institutions. The concept of human rights is broader than what lawyers call "negative" rights—i.e., the right to be free from governmental restraint and discrimination. Human rights, properly defined, include "positive" rights—e.g., the right to health. The United Nations Covenant on Economic, Social and Cultural Rights recognizes this affirmative dimension; it proclaims a right to the enjoyment of the highest attainable standard of physical and mental health (Art. 12.1). Under this positivistic human rights framework, government possesses an obligation, within the constraints of its resources, to provide an environment conducive to the public's health and well-being. The specific responsibilities range from providing a safe blood supply and AIDS education to ensuring access to health care, basic housing, and nutrition. Economic, social, and cultural rights emerge as powerful human rights concerns, particularly in poorer communities in developed and developing countries (Commonwealth Secretariat, 1990).

An expansive view of human rights demonstrates their integral role in safeguarding public health. However, human rights and public health concerns are not always in harmony. International codes do not view all human rights as absolute, and they recognize the possibility of the derogation of rights in limited circumstances, particularly to safeguard public health. As one example, governments may justifiably force individuals to be vaccinated to protect the health of the community. Conflicts between human rights and human health are inevitable, and it is important to understand that trade-offs between rights and health may be necessary.

This book aims to show why human rights are as serious and integral as public health in the fight against the AIDS pandemic. Human rights are critical because (1) all people share an inherent worth and dignity which sometimes transcends even their own desire to be healthy and (2) human rights and public health are fundamentally interconnected.

How should concepts of dignity and the interdependence of human rights and public health affect our thinking and our subsequent approach to the AIDS pandemic? Many people, particularly in poor areas of the world, will never receive the health care and social support that they deserve as human beings. However, it is well within the power of all governments to respect and defend the human rights of their populations. A person living with HIV/AIDS can lead a rewarding life if she is free from governmental coercion or punishment and enjoys respect within her community. A person's right to live her life with dignity and pride, free from restraint, animus, and discrimination, becomes a transcendent value. In the global fight against HIV/AIDS, we must regard the rights of people as highly as we do their health.

A human rights approach is important not only because it promotes respect for individuals, but also because such respect is indispensable to improve public health (International Federation of Red Cross and Red Crescent Societies, François-Xavier Bagnoud Center for Health and Human Rights [IFRC, FXB], 1995). Respecting human rights is the surest way to encourage people to participate in public health programs that offer testing, counseling, education, partner notification, and treatment. It simply is not feasible to *impose* substantial behavioral changes to reduce unprotected sex or sharing of drug injection equipment. It is vitally important to human health that people, communities, and public health programs cooperate. Where governments fail to protect human rights, or worse, where they deprive individuals of rights, government policies are more likely to drive people away from public health programs than to ensure their participation.

Public health thinking is undergoing a transformation. While public health officials have historically exercised compulsory powers to control disease epidemics, modern thinking, particularly in HIV/AIDS, has favored a voluntaristic approach. Public health recommendations at the global, regional, and national level rely on principles of confidentiality, consent, and cooperation (United Nations [UNAIDS], 1996; United Nations, 1996a, 1995c). The clear consensus on this ethic of voluntarism demonstrates that respect for human dignity is essential not simply from a rights perspective, but from a public health perspective.

This book addresses the broad audience of concerned individuals and organizations that seeks to protect the health and human rights of persons living with HIV/AIDS. On a national level, those who should understand and apply human rights principles include governmental organizations (e.g., health ministries), nongovernmental organizations, community-based groups, policymakers, and persons living with HIV/AIDS. The book is designed to help these individuals and organizations worldwide to attain "literacy" in human rights and public health (Mann, Gostin, et al., 1994). This entails understanding the essential concepts, instruments, and language of human rights, as well as the most effective public health strategies for impeding the HIV/AIDS pandemic.

The five chapters herein attempt to explain human rights principles and apply them to AIDS policy. Chapter 1 describes the international system for the promotion and protection of human rights by reviewing the International Bill of Human Rights and the mechanisms designed to implement and enforce the standards developed. Next, the chapter provides a more detailed explanation of human rights with special relevance to health. It concludes with an examination of some of the critical challenges to the evolution of human rights doctrine: the abuse by states of provisions which allow for limitation of rights and other enforcement problems, the question of how to resolve conflicting or competing rights claims, and the issue of universalism versus cultural relativism. The aim of this first chapter is to provide the reader with a basic understanding of the rights framework, its strengths as well as its inherent weaknesses, and a sense of the richness and complexity of human rights doctrine. Advocates and scholars already familiar with human rights may wish to move directly to the discussion of HIV/AIDS and public health that begins in the second chapter.

Chapter 2 discusses the connections between human rights and public health. Public health policies and programs may directly infringe on the human rights of affected individuals. This is most clear in the case of coercive measures, but may also result from voluntary initiatives. Human rights abuses have a direct impact on the health of individuals in the form of immediate and long-term consequences such as death, dismemberment, disfigurement, morbidity, and disability, as well as psychological sequelae. Finally, the promotion of health may require the promotion of the human rights of vulnerable individuals or populations—for example, where this will empower a group, enabling it to take measures to improve its own health. The second section of Chapter 2 illustrates some of the interconnections with reference to international instruments, consensus statements, and guidelines which specifically address the human rights of persons living with HIV/AIDS.

Chapter 3 provides a step-by-step approach to assessing AIDS policies from a human rights perspective. Healthcare professionals and scientists possess many tools with which to evaluate the public health impact of various strategies. Microbiology, virology, immunology, epidemiology, and biostatistics each employ well-developed methods of analysis. Yet public health professionals and community-based organizations often lack the instruments to measure how policies affect the rights of individuals and their communities. This chapter offers a "human rights impact assessment" measure to equip those committed to defending human rights in public health (Gostin, Mann, 1994).

Chapter 4 discusses major areas of AIDS policy and practice around the world. Nations have implemented a wide array of policies in an attempt to reduce the spread of HIV/AIDS. These include prevention and education, casefinding (testing, screening, reporting or notification, and partner notification), compulsory powers (isolation, quarantine, and criminal prosecutions), travel and immigration restrictions, and harm reduction strategies (e.g., needle and syringe exchanges and condom distribution). Chapter 4 examines these policies from a public health and human rights perspective.

The final chapter presents a series of case studies that illustrate key issues in AIDS and human rights. The case studies involve difficult policy and ethical choices: discrimination and the transmission of HIV and tuberculosis in an occupational health care setting; breast-feeding in the least developed countries; and confidentiality and the right of sexual partners to know of potential exposure to HIV. An analysis of the conflicts and possible resolutions helps to show the value of a human rights impact assessment.

This book does not offer easy answers because there are none for the complex AIDS pandemic. Nor does it suggest that the impact on human rights is the only consideration in designing public health policy. But it does argue that human rights need to be treated as seriously as science, medicine, and public health. Policymakers, practitioners, and advocates need to forge new links between human rights and the health of individuals and communities. Incorporating human rights as a global principle in health planning can help revitalize the public health field, renew society's commitment to respect persons, and save lives.

Human Rights and Public Health in the AIDS Pandemic

1

International Human Rights Law in the AIDS Pandemic

THE STRUCTURE OF INTERNATIONAL HUMAN RIGHTS LAW: CODIFICATION, IMPLEMENTATION, ENFORCEMENT

Although human rights and public health present complementary approaches to advancing peoples' well-being, only recently has human rights discourse begun to encompass health-related entitlements. Many reasons exist for this. Perhaps the primary reason, however, involves the evolution of state responsibility for promoting and protecting human rights. Human rights doctrine has always held that "[s]ince human rights and fundamental freedoms are indivisible, the full realization of civil and political rights without the enjoyment of economic, social and cultural rights is impossible" (Proclamation of Teheran, 1968). As the concept of state responsibility for violations developed, debate ensued over the appropriate nature of accountability. The result was a hierarchy of claims, that is, a ranking of rights by enforceability. Because states observe economic and social rights by pursuing certain objectives, rather than by adhering to immediately identifiable standards, rights such as health came to be seen by some as a long-term goal rather than an entitlement. Recent efforts to fully define and analyze the right to health and its relationship to other human rights result from the renewed recognition that all human rights constitute entitlements and are, moreover, inextricably interlinked (Jamar, 1994; Leary, 1994; Mann, Gostin, et al., 1994).

International human rights is a complex and evolving body of law. This chapter sets forth its basic structure, its relevant instruments, and its implementation and enforcement mechanisms. This review is intended not to be comprehensive, but rather to acquaint the reader with the basic concepts of human rights law. A more detailed description will follow of some of the human rights that are most relevant to attaining and advancing individuals' physical and mental well-being. The chapter concludes with a discussion of the issues that continue to influence the development of human rights law.

This chapter seeks to explain the sources of authority in international law for human rights. These sources are indispensable to attaining, advancing, and protecting health.

Understanding them is the first step in recognizing how human rights may promote global strategies to stem the HIV/AIDS pandemic.

Background

The international system to protect human rights grew out of international revulsion at the atrocities committed during World War II. The pre-war international system had focused solely on relations between states; human rights violations that occurred within a country's borders were generally deemed an "internal affair." The horrors of the war exposed the vulnerability of the individual in an international system that was based on state sovereignty and demonstrated the gross inadequacy of previous attempts to protect the victims of war. The violations were recognized as a grave threat to international peace and security and "were linked in the rhetoric of the war and in the plans for peace" (Henkin, 1979). One of the first imperatives of the postwar era was to prevent the recurrence of such egregious affronts to peace and human dignity.

The postwar human rights movement permanently altered the scope of international law (Cassese, 1990). It pierced the veil of national sovereignty and elevated human rights as a matter of international import. The idea that individuals possess inherent rights and freedoms was not new. Recognizing these rights under international law, however, was, as was holding states accountable for violations.

Codification
The UN Charter

In its preamble, the United Nations Charter articulates the international community's determination "to reaffirm faith in fundamental human rights, [and] in the dignity and worth of the human person." One of the central purposes of the United Nations is to achieve international cooperation in "promoting and encouraging respect for human rights and for fundamental freedoms for all without distinction" (UN Charter, Art. 1). The Charter, as a binding treaty, pledges member states to promote:

> Higher standards of living, full employment, and conditions of economic and social progress and development; solutions of international economic, social, health, and related problems; international cultural and educational cooperation; and, universal respect for, and observance of, human rights and fundamental freedoms for all without distinction as to race, sex, language, or religion. (UN Charter, Art. 55, 56).

Although somewhat amorphous in that it requires only "promotional" activities, the statement nonetheless recognizes a connection between basic needs and freedom from want, and respect for and observance of fundamental civil and political rights.

The International Bill of Human Rights

The Universal Declaration of Human Rights (UDHR), adopted in 1948, built upon the UN Charter's promise by identifying specific rights and freedoms that deserve promotion and protection. The UDHR's adoption set the stage for a treaty-based scheme to promote and protect human rights, realized in 1966 when the International Covenant on Civil and Political Rights (ICCPR) and the International Covenant on Economic, Social and Cultural Rights (ICESCR) were adopted. After ratification or accession by at least thirty-five member countries, the Covenants entered into force in 1976. Together, the Universal Declaration and the two International Covenants on Human Rights (along with the subsequently enhanced Optional Protocol to the ICCPR) constitute the International Bill of Human Rights, the backbone of the international human rights system.

The Universal Declaration of Human Rights

The UDHR, approved by forty-eight states with eight abstentions, was the organized international community's first attempt to establish "a common standard of achievement for all peoples and all nations" to promote human rights. The document proclaims the equal significance of civil and political rights and economic, social, and cultural rights. The Declaration's thirty articles are based upon the principle that "[a]ll human beings are born free and equal in dignity and rights" (Art. 1). The rights set forth are to be respected without discrimination and include the right to life, liberty, and security of person; the prohibition of slavery, torture, and cruel, inhuman, or degrading treatment; the right to an effective judicial remedy; the prohibition of arbitrary arrest, detention, and exile; the right to be presumed innocent until proven guilty and to receive a fair trial; freedom from arbitrary interference with one's privacy, family, or home; freedom of movement and residence; freedom of conscience, religion, and expression; freedom of association; and the right to participate in the government of one's country.

The UDHR characterizes economic, social, and cultural rights as "indispensable for [a person's] dignity and the development of his personality" (Art. 22). Set forth in Articles 22 through 27, these rights include the right to social security; the right to work, to receive equal pay for equal work, and to remuneration ensuring "an existence worthy of human dignity"; the right to education; and the right to share in the cultural life of the community and "to share in scientific advancement and its benefits." Article 25 of the UDHR expressly recognizes a claim to health:

> Everyone has the right to a standard of living adequate for the health and well-being of himself and his family, including food, clothing, housing and medical care and necessary social services, and the right to security in the event of unemployment, sickness, disability, widowhood, old age or other lack of livelihood in circumstances beyond his control.

Interestingly, during the drafting of the UDHR, the emphasis shifted from a direct focus on the right to health to its current focus on the economic necessities essential to achieving human health. The original draft declared that "[e]veryone, without distinction as to economic and social conditions, has the right to the preservation of his health" through the appropriate standard of food, clothing, housing, and medical care. This language was subsequently deleted in favor of the "right to a standard of living necessary for health and general well-being" (United Nations Yearbook, 1948). The difference is subtle, but the current document appears to emphasize economic policies that will ensure a minimal standard of health, as opposed to a range of policies designed to protect the community's health.

The Universal Declaration has largely fulfilled the promise of its preamble, becoming the "common standard" for evaluating respect for human rights. Although it was not promulgated to legally bind member states, its key provisions have so often been applied and accepted that they are now widely considered to have attained the status of customary international law. The Universal Declaration embodies what is meant by "human rights" in the international community, and it has inspired successive generations of legally binding human rights instruments.

The International Bill of Human Rights recognizes individuals' duty to the community, creates absolute (nonderogable) rights, and outlines criteria for the limitation of other rights.

In acknowledging the individual's duty to the community, Article 29 of the Universal Declaration states simply: "Everyone has duties to the community in which alone the free and full development of his personality is possible." The drafters, however, offered little guidance regarding the meaning. Logically, individuals' duties must include respect for the human rights of others, including the right to health. Individuals, therefore, have a responsibility to behave in ways that will not harm others, for example, by not exposing their sexual or needle-sharing partners to the risk of HIV infection. In December 1995, the World AIDS Day theme was "shared rights, shared responsibilities," suggesting that all members of a community have a responsibility to respect and protect their own and other's rights and health.

Certain rights are so essential to human dignity and well-being as to be absolute (e.g., the right to be free from torture). Absolute rights can never be abrogated, regardless of the justification; international human rights law permits no exceptions. In some sense, international law provides a "stopping rule" that will not countenance acts which are so abhorrent to humankind that they can never be justified, even for an ostensibly greater good.

Other human rights, however, may be limited in certain situations. Article 29 of the Universal Declaration counsels that such restrictions must be "determined by law solely for the purpose of securing due recognition and respect for the rights and freedoms of others and of meeting the just requirements of morality, public order and the general welfare in a democratic society." Generally, restrictions on human rights must be (1) *prescribed by law in a democratic society*—based upon the legislature's thoughtful consideration and (2) *necessary to protect a valued social goal*—promoting a compelling public interest (e.g., safety or health). Balancing individual rights against larger social concerns demands an acute sensitivity to the nature of the burden imposed on the individual and the limits permitted by human rights law.

The International Covenants on human rights

Given the inclusiveness of the Universal Declaration, the drafters' initial plan was apparently to craft a comprehensive human rights treaty. Fairly early in the process, however, the drafters concluded that implementing civil and political rights called for one approach, while economic, social, and cultural rights demanded another. The solution was to draft parallel but separate instruments. Nonetheless, both Covenants reflect the Universal Declaration's dictate that the highest aspirations of humanity may be achieved by realizing civil and political, as well as economic, social, and cultural rights (ICCPR preamble; ICESCR preamble). The Covenants share certain substantive protections, namely, the right to self-determination (Art. 1) and prohibition of discrimination (Art. 2). In addition, both Covenants recognize the right to form trade unions (ICCPR, Art. 22; ICESCR, Art. 8) and the family's right to special protections (ICCPR, Art. 23; ICESCR, Art. 10); each Covenant develops these rights somewhat differently, though, reflecting their differing foci.

The International Covenant on Civil and Political Rights (ICCPR) includes most, but not all, of the civil and political rights addressed in the UDHR. Additionally, the document recognizes rights such as that of ethnic, religious, and linguistic minorities to enjoy their own culture, practice their own religion, and use their own language. Furthermore, the ICCPR requires that persons deprived of liberty be treated humanely and respected for their inherent dignity and accords the minor the protection "required by his status as a minor."

The International Covenant on Economic, Social and Cultural Rights (ICESCR) greatly expands upon the UDHR's treatment of these rights. Sections of the ICESCR form the foundation for "positive rights," that is, those requiring proactivity from the state. Such affirmative rights include family protection, an adequate standard of living, and education. Article 12, for instance, requires a state to undertake certain defined steps to meet "the right of everyone to the highest attainable standard of physical and mental health." The steps include:

> (a) The provision for the reduction of the stillbirth-rate and of infant mortality and for the healthy development of the child; (b) The improvement of all aspects of environmental and industrial hygiene; (c) The prevention, treatment and control of epidemic, endemic, occupational and other diseases; (d) The creation of conditions which would assure to all medical service and medical attention in the event of sickness.

The ICESCR's *traveaux preparatoires* suggest that the right to health was largely formulated on the principles of the World Health Organization's Constitution (although several principles originally considered were later deleted). From a human rights perspective, the right as articulated prioritizes the claims of certain groups, such as infants, children, and persons at risk of disease. From a health perspective, the Article delineates concrete steps and establishes a measure of accountability through the use of specific indicators, such as reduction in stillbirths and infant mortality.

In their treatment of permissible limitations, the two Covenants diverge. The ICCPR recognizes that certain rights are so fundamental as to be absolute and proscribes any derogation of them. Nonderogable rights include the right to life (Art. 6); freedom from torture and from cruel, inhuman, or degrading treatment or punishment (Art. 7); freedom from slavery or involuntary servitude (Art. 8); freedom from imprisonment based solely on failure to fulfill a contractual obligation (Art. 11); freedom from ex post facto criminal provisions (Art. 15); the right to recognition as a person before the law (Art. 16); and freedom of thought, conscience, and religion (Art. 18).

The ICCPR states that other rights may be justifiably limited under certain prescribed conditions. For example, limitations may be permissible "in time of public emergency which threatens the life of the nation" but only "to the extent strictly required by the exigencies of the situation, provided that such measures are not applied in a discriminatory manner and are not inconsistent with their other obligations under international law" (Art. 4.1). Several other provisions set forth the possibility of limitations. For instance, freedom of movement may justifiably be limited where restrictions are "provided for by law, are necessary to protect national security, public order, public health or morals or the rights and freedoms of others" (Art 12.3). Similarly, freedom to manifest one's religion (Art. 18.3), to exchange information, expression, and to hold opinions (Art. 19.3), to assemble peaceably (Art. 21), and to associate with others (Art. 22.2) may all be restricted on comparable grounds.

The ICESCR, on the other hand, states: "[T]he state may subject such rights only to such limitations as are determined by law only in so far as this may be compatible with the nature of these rights and solely for the purpose of promoting the general welfare in a democratic society" (Art. 4).

Standards of Implementation

The decision to draft parallel international conventions reflected the view that no single system of implementation could appropriately address both sets of rights. Not surprisingly, the instruments differ in how they are to be effectuated. The implementation schemes try to account for the relative differences in the time, effort, and resources necessary to achieve each set of rights. The ICCPR requires states "to respect and to ensure," or, in other words, to guarantee their citizens immediate and full enjoyment of the rights enumerated (Art. 2). Many of the ICCPR's provisions require the state to refrain from certain conduct. Theoretically, the state can fulfill this duty through legislative measures, without a substantial investment of additional resources.

In contrast, the ICESCR holds as its goal the "progressive realization" of the rights and recognizes the need for international assistance to enable some countries to realize these rights (United Nations, 1991b). The ICESCR requires:

Each State Party to the present Covenant undertakes to take steps, individually and through international assistance and cooperation, especially economic and technical, to the maximum of its available resources, with a view to achieving progressively the full realization of the rights recognized in the present Covenant by all appropriate means, including particularly the adoption of legislative measures. (Art. 2)

Many ICESCR provisions detail a list of steps for realizing these rights, as with the right to health (ICESCR, Art. 12). This emphasis on incremental achievement acknowledges that many of these rights require an ample investment of human and material resources and recognizes that states occupy disparate levels of economic, social, educational, and infrastructure development. In regard to the right to health, for instance, the postwar period found many developed countries with a fairly comprehensive public health system in place. In contrast, during the same era in the developing world, even the most rudimentary state-supported health institutions and programs were often unavailable outside of major cities. These countries faced an overwhelming number of problems (e.g., training health care providers and providing adequate financial and material resources to build, equip, staff, and operate programs and facilities). To have expected countries to accomplish these tasks quickly would have been unrealistic. Even now, some countries might never achieve these steps without international assistance.

Certain economic, social, and cultural rights are particularly difficult to define and measure. The lack of precise standards may not be as troubling where states are only required to move toward a goal rather than realize it. The lack of a clear and comprehensive definition of the right to health (Art. 12), however, should not preclude countries from initiating measures to improve their populations' health.

Although the implementation provisions of the ICESCR are less concrete and immediate than those of the ICCPR, the ICESCR requires specific compliance. Each state party is required to "take steps" immediately, particularly economic and technical ones, toward fully achieving the rights. Moreover, the steps taken must utilize available resources and, where necessary, rely upon international assistance and cooperation.

Enforcement Mechanisms

The two Covenants differ sharply in the measures they establish to encourage or enforce compliance. The ICCPR contains by far the more sophisticated apparatus, a complex system of reporting, monitoring, investigating, and adjudicating complaints.

The ICCPR established the Human Rights Committee (HRC) to oversee compliance by the "State Parties" who adopt it. The HRC has four functions: (1) at public meetings, it examines reports submitted by State Parties documenting their implementation of Covenant provisions; (2) it issues "general comments" to clarify certain provisions; (3) it investigates interstate complaints where both states accept its jurisdiction; and (4) it examines individuals' complaints against states that have adopted the Optional Protocol to the ICCPR. The Optional Protocol empowers private persons to seek redress for Covenant violations from the HRC but is only available for use against states that have ratified it. The Optional Protocol binds approximately half of the states that are parties to the Covenant. The enforcement system involves not only the Human Rights Committee but also national and international nongovernmental organizations (NGOs). These organizations have become instrumental in identifying and investigating civil and political rights violations worldwide (Hannum, 1986).

Beyond reporting, few mechanisms exist to monitor or enforce the ICESCR's provisions. Member states periodically report to the UN Economic and Social Council (ECOSOC) regarding measures adopted and progress made. ECOSOC also receives information from various specialized UN agencies, particularly the World Health Organization (WHO). NGOs have been less active in monitoring economic, social, and cultural rights compared to civil and political rights. Furthermore, little jurisprudence has developed on regional, national, or international levels concerning economic, social, and cultural rights (Steiner, 1991). Increasingly, however, world attention is turning to issues of economic, social, and cultural rights. The Economic and Social Council is actively seeking new ways to evaluate these rights as a step toward effectuating their status as rights, while facilitating their definition, implementation, and evaluation.

Special rapporteurs (reporters) also monitor and report findings to UN bodies on particular issues involving international human rights law. These investigators research specific topics or survey certain countries or regions (see United Nations, 1995d, 1993, 1992, 1991).

Some regional entities may afford redress for human rights violations. Regional human rights charters often establish commissions to oversee the enforcement of their provisions. For example, the African Charter on Human and Peoples' Rights set up an elected, eleven-member commission which attempts to resolve complaints through negotiation rather than adversarial debate. The European Convention for the Protection of Human Rights and Fundamental Freedoms (ECHR) established both the European Commission on Human Rights and the European Court of Human Rights (ECHR signed 1950, entered into force, 1953, Art. 19).

Protections against human rights violations exist at the international, regional, national, and local levels. Enforcement relies heavily upon the voluntary compliance and self-policing efforts of individual countries, which usually perceive some self-interest in such actions. In addition, enforcement is closely related to the degree of international pressure exerted on the offending country by international and regional governmental and nongovernmental organizations, other nations, national organizations, and even individuals. In this aspect, human rights resemble other areas of international law (Bilder, 1986).

People who wish to lodge a human rights complaint, or seek to influence policy, usually begin at the local or national level if an appropriate forum exists. Individuals tend to have more realistic opportunities to effect change in their own communities and countries, where they are most familiar with legal and democratic processes. Some international mechanisms, moreover, require claimants to first exhaust national remedies before these procedures may be triggered. If no effective remedies exist at the national or local level, or all have been exhausted, international remedies may represent the only recourse.

Effective advocacy, locally or nationally, requires a full understanding and strict adherence to a particular state's enforcement system. Many levels of entry exist, including human rights commissions, independent tribunals, and courts. Contacting a public official, nongovernmental organization, or community leader may lead to meaningful information and assistance, and perhaps to speedier redress.

Nongovernmental organizations (NGOs) are invaluable sources of information about state and local practices. Furthermore, they may help in forwarding individuals' complaints to formal international bodies. Representatives of NGOs frequently attend HRC meetings, query members, and apprise members of (often well-documented) concerns. Such groups are growing in number and are among the most dynamic partners in implementing and enforcing human rights (Picken, 1985; Shestack, 1978). HIV/AIDS-related issues continue to increase the importance of NGO participation, monitoring, and overall contribution to human rights and health. The Joint United Nations Programme on HIV/AIDS (UNAIDS), founded in 1996, is the first program of the United Nations system to include NGO representation on its governing body (United Nations [UNAIDS], 1996b).

Individuals and groups may improve state human rights practices through avenues outside of the formal legal structure. Two types of informal mechanisms are publicity and direct action. Both may effect policy changes and help specific individuals. For interstate complaints, publicity is likely to be more effective than individual appeals, although the latter may, in certain circumstances, strengthen state efforts.

To date, formal enforcement tools on the international and regional levels have not been effectively wielded to combat HIV/AIDS-related human rights violations. Existing human rights treaty bodies and UNAIDS potentially play a significant role in monitoring compliance with human rights standards in the context of HIV/AIDS. The Commission on Human Rights has recommended that United Nations bodies dealing with human rights monitoring and enforcement adopt concrete means to review protection of HIV-related human rights as part of their specific mandates and procedures (United Nations 1996a).

Advocates for persons with HIV have been successful in securing redress through informal channels and through formal legal mechanisms at the national level. For example, a court order in the United States closed the detention camp at Guantanamo Bay, Cuba, used to imprison HIV-infected Haitians seeking political asylum. A French court provided redress for people who contracted HIV through transfusions from an inadequately screened blood supply. Publicity curtailed unethical research on HIV-infected children in Romania.

In addition, to reduce the likelihood of transmission, advocates have employed publicity to educate populations about high-risk behaviors and practices. Using the media, advocates have pressured governments to develop and fund AIDS education, prevention, and treatment efforts in many parts of the world.

Further Developments in the Protection of Human Rights

Additional human rights instruments

Scores of treaties, promulgated by an array of sources too numerous to catalogue, have amplified the UN Charter and the International Bill of Rights to address specific human rights abuses (Table 1-1). For example, the International Labor Organization (ILO) has developed a panoply of human rights instruments and enforcement mechanisms. As of 1993, the ILO had promulgated 174 binding conventions and 181 recommendations regarding employment and labor issues. The ILO Constitution recognizes that labor is not a commodity to be traded like other goods. It also affirms the right of all human beings—irrespective of race, creed, or sex—to pursue their material well-being and spiritual development under conditions of freedom, dignity, economic security, and equal opportunity (Widdows, 1993).

Article 12 of the ICESCR has been augmented by or spawned additional international legal standards regarding the right to health. The norms, however, are dispersed throughout a variety of instruments. Many aspects of international cooperation implicitly or explicitly impact human health. Subsequently, concern for health is evidenced in instruments that address human rights, development, the environment, occupational health, health protection in armed conflict, and countless others (Tomasevski, 1995; see Chapter 2, Aids Specific Documents, reviewing nonbinding instruments and guidelines with special reference to HIV/AIDS).

Regional human rights systems

Regional human rights systems uniquely contribute to the promotion and protection of human rights. These systems are based on their own constitutive instruments and

Table 1-1 Selected Documents Addressing Specific Abuses of Human Rights

The United Nations Convention on the Prevention and Punishment of the Crime of Genocide (1951)

The United Nations International Convention on the Elimination of Racial Discrimination (1969)

The International Convention on the Suppression and Punishment of Apartheid (1973)

The Helsinki Accord (1975)

The Convention on the Elimination of All Forms of Discrimination Against Women (1979)

The United Nations Declaration on the Elimination of Intolerance and Discrimination Based on Religion or Belief (1981)

The United Nations Declaration on the Right of Peoples to Peace (1984)

The Convention Against Torture and Other Cruel, Inhuman or Degrading Treatment or Punishment (1984)

The United Nations Declaration on the Right to Development (1986)

The United Nations Declaration on the Rights of Persons with Disability (1987)

The United Nations Declaration on the Rights of Persons with Mental Illness (1991)

have produced a range of comprehensive implementation and enforcement machinery. The regional systems complement the global UN system and possess the potential for specialized human rights action that is swifter and more contextually responsive than that on the international plane. In some cases, regional systems offer stronger enforcement mechanisms. Moreover, regional mechanisms may be more accessible to those who seek to promote or to vindicate human rights in their own countries. However, the existence of practical remedies and the actual availability of relief depends on cooperation of member states. In areas experiencing civil or international unrest, governments may be unable or unwilling to respond to human rights issues raised by regional organizations.

European Agreements. In 1950, the Council of Europe proposed the European Convention on Human Rights and Fundamental Freedoms (ECHR) to promote civil and political rights. In 1953, the ECHR was ratified by every state in the Council of Europe and has since been complemented by a series of additional protocols. ECHR members recognize the European Commission of Human Rights' automatic jurisdiction over complaints filed by other states, and by individuals where the state involved acknowledges the Commission's jurisdiction. The European Court of Human Rights exercises jurisdiction over states which expressly declare their acceptance thereof. As with the Inter-American system (see below), only the Commission and states may bring a case before the European Court. The European Social Charter, which entered into force in 1965, is an indispensable guide to economic, social, and cultural rights in Europe. The European system has produced the largest and most frequently cited body of regional human rights jurisprudence.

The African Charter on Human and Peoples' Rights. The African Charter on Human and Peoples' Rights (1986) mandates that governments prohibit discriminatory conduct. Originally adopted by the Organization of African Unity (OAU), by 1986, the African Charter had been ratified by more than thirty states. The Charter is more extensive than other regional conventions; in addition to protecting Africans' political, civil, economic, social, and cultural rights, it addresses the communal responsibility of individuals toward one another and the state. The African Commission on Human and Peoples' Rights monitors adherence to the Charter. The Commission conducts promotional activities, sets standards, and processes individual complaints of violations.

Inter-American System. The Inter-American system of human rights encompasses the Charter of the Organization of American States, the American Declaration on the Rights and Duties of Man (1948), and the American Convention on Human Rights (ACHR). The ACHR, which came into force in 1978, is the preeminent legally binding human rights document in the Americas. The Convention guarantees the protection of civil and political rights. The Optional Protocol on Economic Social and Cultural Rights has yet to enter into effect.

The Inter-American Commission on Human Rights is automatically authorized to process individual complaints of violations. It exercises Convention-based jurisdiction over states parties thereto and Charter-based jurisdiction over other member states through the American Declaration. Furthermore, the ACHR established the Inter-American Court of Human Rights, which is empowered to exercise both advisory and compulsory jurisdiction. It may invoke the latter, however, only where Convention parties have expressly accepted it.

Permanent Arab Commission on Human Rights. Founded in 1945, the League of Arab States established in 1968 the Permanent Arab Commission on Human Rights as one of its contributions to the International Human Rights Year. Each League member is represented on the Commission, which drafts human rights agreements to submit to the Council of the Arab League. In addition, the Commission may submit its own suggestions to the Council (Robertson, Merrills, 1989).

HUMAN RIGHTS WITH SPECIAL RELEVANCE TO PUBLIC HEALTH AND HIV/AIDS

Health policymakers and practitioners need not know in detail the many international declarations, covenants, resolutions, implementing standards, and enforcement mechanisms. However, general familiarity with these instruments and systems can assist people in more effectively fighting the AIDS pandemic. To this end, this section explores core human rights principles and considers each in the context of the HIV/AIDS pandemic. Understanding of, and sensitivity to, these principles will enable health care professionals, public health officials, nongovernmental organizations, persons with AIDS, and others to identify human rights abuses, develop effective public health policies, and advocate for a more humane society.

Civil and Political Rights

Right to life

International law defends the most fundamental of all human rights: the right to life. Article 3 of the Universal Declaration proclaims: "Everyone has the right to life." The ICCPR specifies an "inherent right to life . . . protected by law. No one shall be arbitrarily deprived of life" (Art. 6.1). The right to life is an essential condition for the enjoyment of all human rights (United Nations, 1984, pp. 39–45). The UN General Assembly has called for cooperation by inter- and nongovernmental organizations to ensure that scientific and technological progress will be channeled to promote peace and to benefit humankind (United Nations, 1984, p. 38).

The United Nation's proposal to harness science and technology to aid humankind involves public health policy. Scientific advances have enabled public health workers to track the course of disease epidemics, target prevention strategies, improve treatment, and prevent illness through vaccination. But scientific knowledge alone is not enough; implementation and resources are required. The HIV/AIDS pandemic is more than fifteen years old, and many countries have yet to implement universal screening of blood and other tissues because they lack trained personnel, resources, and testing kits. Similarly, an effective hepatitis B vaccine has existed for over a decade, but is not used in most developing countries where hepatitis B remains a significant cause of morbidity and mortality. Such failures to employ existing technologies result in preventable illness and death.

If science and technology are to better humankind, scientific advances must be made available to poorer countries. This obligation becomes more compelling as the international community conducts clinical trials for HIV/AIDS vaccines and treatment. Even safe and effective vaccines and treatments will challenge the global community. The theme of the XI International Conference on AIDS (Vancouver, Canada, July 7–12, 1996), "One World, One Hope," focused on the need to eliminate the current inequities in the distribution of the benefits of important HIV/AIDS research. Countries that suffer the greatest burden of disease—but possess the fewest resources—must be assured the ability to purchase and distribute vaccines or treatment.

Freedom from inhuman and degrading treatment

Article 5 of the Universal Declaration of Human Rights states: "No one shall be subjected to torture or to cruel, inhuman or degrading treatment or punishment." The International Covenant on Civil and Political Rights (Art. 7) contains a similar prohibition but phrases it more as an entitlement: "All persons deprived of their liberty shall be treated with humanity and respect for the inherent dignity of the human person" (Art. 10). The prohibition of torture and cruel, inhuman, or degrading treatment is a fundamental, nonderogable right (ICCPR, Art. 4.2; Declaration on the Protection of All Persons from Being Subjected to Torture and Other Cruel, Inhuman or Degrading Treatment or Punishment, 1975). Governments, therefore, may not subject persons with HIV or AIDS to inhuman and degrading treatment even if purportedly in the community's interests.

Human rights organizations (e.g., the World Health Organization, the Council for International Organizations of the Medical Sciences [CIOMS], the World Medical Assembly, and the General Assembly of the United Nations) have roundly condemned the participation of health care professionals in acts constituting torture or cruel, inhuman, or degrading treatment (Principles of Medical Ethics, 1982).

The Right to Humane, Dignified, and Professional Treatment. Article 5 of the Universal Declaration of Human Rights guarantees that persons deprived of their liberty "shall be treated with humanity and respect for the inherent dignity of the human person." Squalid conditions of confinement in a health care facility or prison may constitute inhuman or degrading treatment. Conditions such as unjustified or grossly humiliating mental or physical deprivations would likely violate this right (*A. v. United Kingdom*, 1980; *B. v. United Kingdom*, 1981).

Statutes, policies, programs, or practices that impair or deny liberty to persons with HIV infection or AIDS should be evaluated by the standard of humane, dignified, and professional treatment provided to persons in confinement. Persons deprived of liberty to promote public health are entitled, at a minimum, to safe, healthful, and humane conditions and medical treatment. This means that the situation and setting must be consistent with the purpose of confinement. Persons convicted of criminal offenses must have decent health care, safe and sanitary conditions, proper nutrition, and an appropriate range of recreational and other privileges within the prison system. This includes, for example, the right not to be secluded for extended periods and the right to be protected from physical harm such as violence or infectious disease (e.g., tuberculosis). Persons confined under public health or mental health powers must be placed in a health care facility suitable to their needs. Health status alone cannot justify criminal confinement. Thus, persons with HIV infection who are subject to isolation, quarantine, or civil commitment may not be confined as a punitive measure. These persons are entitled to safe, humane, and healthful conditions.

Right to security[1]

Informed Consent. The right to personal security necessitates that individuals retain control over their bodies. To realize this right, individuals must remain free to voluntarily accept or refuse physical intrusions, even when the purpose is benign. The doctrine of voluntary consent to medical testing, treatment, or research, which much of the international community endorses, may be seen as arising from the right to security of person. International resolutions—ranging from the Nuremberg Code, the Declaration of Helsinki, and the Geneva Convention to modern codes on research ethics such as the Council of International Organizations of Medical Sciences (CIOMS) Guidelines on Biomedical and Epidemiological Research (1991, 1993)—widely recognize a patient or research subject's right to grant or withhold consent. A govern-

---

1. We chose to discuss the doctrine of informed consent under the right to security of the person instead of the right to self-determination. The first Article of each of the International Covenants on human rights proclaims: "All peoples have the right to self-determination. By virtue of that right they freely determine their political status and freely pursue their economic, social and cultural development." In 1952, the General Assembly recognized self-determination as a "prerequisite to the full enjoyment of all fundamental human rights" (United Nations, 1984, pp. 31–33). The United Nations has construed this right as a collective right of peoples and countries to be free and to have control over their destiny—implying political self-rule or self-governance. The right, however, also belongs to each individual. A fundamental respect for autonomy undergirds the right of individual self-determination. Each person possesses an inalienable right to make decisions without undue coercion (Beauchamp, Childress, 1994).

ment may restrict that right only if indispensable to achieving a compelling public health interest.

Individuals cannot give meaningful consent without adequate information about the nature, purpose, and potential adverse effects of the procedure. Appropriate and sufficient information enables an autonomous person to carefully weigh the risks and benefits and to thoughtfully choose among alternatives. Under robust conceptions of informed consent, individuals must be given full and objective information. Moreover, the person must be competent to grasp the nature and consequences of her decision, and to consent freely. Only when competent persons make uncoerced choices, based on full information, can they truly exercise their right to security of person. Security, then, requires information, competency, and a voluntary assent to intervention absent undue influence, duress, or coercion.

Some claim that the doctrine of informed consent is a Northern/Western construct with little relevance for non-Western societies. Many countries, particularly in the South and East, conceptualize health as a collective responsibility, about which the family and community, not the individual, properly make decisions (Christakis, 1988; Ajayi, 1980; Ekunwe, Kessel, 1984; Hall, 1989).

This cultural difference does not negate the need for informed consent. "While consent procedures must be adapted to accommodate cultural mores, there must always be a requirement for consent from the individual" (World Health Organization, 1989h).

Some critics argue that informed consent is impractical in populations with high illiteracy rates. Yet, comprehensible information can be presented consistent with reading abilities, language, custom, and culture. Moreover, informed consent and strong familial and societal ties are not mutually exclusive. Deference to family and community leaders, and responsibility to society, do not preclude a person from providing his or her own consent (Ankrah, Gostin, 1994).

The Council of International Organizations of Medical Sciences (CIOMS, 1991) suggests that health care professionals are ethically obligated to obtain consent on three levels, when culturally appropriate. The *informed consent of the individual* is critical. In some cultures, *permission of a trusted family member or elder* is also advisable. When the intervention may impact the entire community (as in epidemiologic research), a *community consensus* from an appropriate representative is important. As cumulative ethical obligations, the successive concepts of individual consent, permission, and consensus should be evaluated within the context of international human rights and local cultural norms (Gostin, 1991).

The nation of Gambia employs an effective model of consent, permission, and consensus. Hall (1989) characterizes the system as a hierarchical chain that links the government, the chief of the district, and the head of the village. Village meetings inform people about potential research studies, and each individual votes whether to participate.

Privacy. Privacy, although a highly complex concept, can be defined as the right of individuals to limit access by others to some aspect of their person (Allen, 1987). Privacy is explicitly protected in Article 12 of the Universal Declaration of Human Rights (1948). Article 12 ensures an individual's right to protection from "arbitrary interference with his privacy, family, home or correspondence." The concept of privacy extends not only to private acts and the physical space within one's home, but also to personal information, including health information. The International Covenant of Civil and Political Rights proscribes both arbitrary and unlawful interference with privacy (Art. 17). Therefore, intentional or negligent disclosures of personal information without the person's consent may constitute a breach of privacy. By divulging deeply private aspects of one's personal or family life, breaches of privacy undermine one's integrity.

Confidentiality. Confidentiality refers to the patient's right to expect that health care professionals will not disclose personal health information without the person's consent. The right to confidentiality embraces intimate matters, such as sexual relationships, illicit drug use, and health status, that a patient might discuss with a health care professional.

Confidentiality serves several important purposes in health care. It promotes human dignity by protecting intimate information, encourages and preserves trust between health care professionals or healers and patients, and increases the efficacy of public health programs that depend on voluntary cooperation to effect lasting behavioral changes (Gostin, 1995). Confidentiality also promotes fully voluntary blood donations to meet a country's needs.

Different cultures define the scope of privacy and confidentiality differently. In Africa, for instance, tradition may dictate that disease and death are viewed as a family or community, rather than an individual, issue. If a person becomes infected with a disease such as HIV/AIDS, the head of the family may decide whether, and from whom, to seek advice or treatment. Even here, however, some matters may be kept confidential. A family may maintain secrecy if it does not want others to know that one of its members has a chronic illness or genetic defect. In these situations, traditional healers and diviners do not disclose the nature of the illness except to those family members, elders, or clansmen who are privy to group secrets. Others who have gone through appropriate rituals may also share in the information. In this way, the confidentiality of individual health matters is preserved, while the family is shielded from ostracism, isolation, or stigmatization (Ankrah, Gostin, 1994).

Some commentators have described the concept of "shared confidentiality" in Africa. Shared confidentiality rests on the tradition of informing relatives, and often neighbors, about important situations. Those who are apprised of the information keep it from those outside the group. Thus, a group shares the burden of an individual's illness but mutually agrees to ensure the person's privacy. While an infected person is healthy, shared confidentiality cannot properly be breached. But when a person becomes ill, family members and community elders should be informed because the person may benefit from the community's support, particularly in village settings (Commonwealth Secretariat, 1990).

Although the scope of individual privacy may vary culturally, the core principle does not: An individual may control the disclosure of personal information. To deny such control is, in many situations, contrary to the privacy principles articulated in the UDHR. Although society and culture will likely influence an individual's decision, tradition need not always govern. Cultures may prioritize the role of family, community, or religious leaders in health care decisions, but tradition should not displace the individual's ultimate right to control this information.

Right to Know. Although confidentiality is critical in both health care and public health, it may at times conflict with other legal and ethical claims. Many scholars treat the right to confidentiality as pliable when its protection poses a significant risk of serious injury to others. An identifiable person who faces a significant risk may possess a right to information that, under other circumstances, would be confidential. For example, a person with HIV infection has a privacy right to withhold disclosure of his or her serological status. However, a person who is at significant risk of infection (e.g., a current sexual or needle-sharing partner) may legitimately claim a right to this information. If the risk of harm is great and the knowledge of serological status can reduce or eliminate the risk, a claim of a "right to know" is strong. In contrast, a low risk (e.g., a doctor treats a person with HIV/AIDS using universal precautions) or a lack of consequence on health outcomes (e.g., a sex partner properly uses a condom) weakens the claim for the right to know.

Nondiscrimination

The principles of equality and nondiscrimination underlie the purpose of the United Nations and form the foundation for key human rights instruments. Article 56 of the United Nations Charter contains a pledge by all member states to promote respect for human rights and fundamental freedoms for all, regardless of race, sex, language, or religion. The Universal Declaration of Human Rights (1948) states:

> All human beings are born free and equal in dignity and rights. They are endowed with reason and conscience and should act towards one another in a spirit of brotherhood. Everyone is entitled to all the rights and freedoms set forth in this Declaration, without distinction of any kind, such as race, color, sex, language, religion, political or other opinion, national or social origin, property, birth or other status (Art. 1, 2).

The International Covenant on Economic, Social and Cultural Rights (ICESCR) and the International Covenant on Civil and Political Rights (ICCPR) affirm in nearly identical passages principles of equality and nondiscrimination. Both call upon state parties to protect Covenant rights without discrimination as to "race, color, sex, language, religion, political or other opinion, national or social origin, property, birth or other status." Each Covenant reaffirms the equal right of men and women to enjoy and exercise the rights protected (ICESCR; ICCPR, Art. 2, 3).

Discrimination can be defined as any form of differential treatment or classification. It occurs in a multitude of circumstances, not all of which are unethical or unlawful. Therefore, one must identify which types of discrimination are prohibited by international human rights law. Guided by jurisprudence of the European Court of Human Rights and the United Nations Human Rights Committee, the Gambian Minister of Justice, Hassan B. Jallow, distinguished permissible differential treatment from prohibited discrimination: Discrimination is legally permissible only when it is based on reasonable and objective criteria and is morally justified by a compelling need (Jallow, 1991).

Equal administration of justice is an essential corollary of the nondiscrimination principle. The Universal Declaration claims: "Everyone is entitled in full equality to a fair and public hearing by an independent and impartial tribunal, in the determination of his rights and obligations and of any criminal charge against him" (Art. 10). A number of instruments include provisions on the equal administration of justice (e.g., ICCPR, Declaration and Convention on the Elimination of All Forms of Racial Discrimination, and the Declarations and Conventions on the Rights of Women).

Some documents target specific types of discrimination such as race, sex, or religion. Governments can rarely, if ever, justify unequal treatment based on intrinsic personal characteristics which do not affect a person's abilities, strengths, and inherent dignity.

Discrimination and Health. Invidious government discrimination perpetuates poor health in some communities. Policies like apartheid that maintained a segregated health system resulted in a higher incidence of preventable disease and infant mortality, and a lower life expectancy among disadvantaged groups.

Discrimination against women is particularly pervasive and adversely affects their health. Women living in poor or rural areas of many countries suffer from malnutrition in greater numbers than do men. In addition, compared to men, women often receive less health care for common problems (Chen, Souza, 1981; Ravindran, 1986). When governments fail to recognize the differing health care needs of men and women, they discriminate against women (Cook, 1992; Gruskin, 1995). To illustrate, a lack of family planning, obstetric, and perinatal services inordinately affects women and is strongly associated with elevated levels of preventable infant and maternal mortality. Exclusion of women from clinical trials may constitute a subtler form of discrimination by denying women equal benefit from ongoing scientific inquiry. Routinely barring women from clinical trials results in less knowledge about diseases in, or drugs for, women, and less data regarding their safe and effective treatment.

Discrimination in health care occurs globally, in varying forms. It includes discrimination because of gender, ethnicity, or social class; stigmatization due to certain diseases; and denial of access to treatment, care, or research. Acknowledging these persistent problems, the Commission on Human Rights (United Nations, 1989c) concludes that "all human rights must apply to all patients without exception and that non-discrimination in the field of health should apply to all people and in all circumstances." In their role as interpreters of human rights language and norms, the Commission on Human Rights and its Sub-Commission on Prevention of Discrimination and Protection of Minorities has confirmed that under existing international law, discrimination on the basis of "other status" is prohibited, which includes health status and infection or perception of infection with HIV/AIDS (United Nations, 1995a, b, 1996a).

Freedom of opinion and expression

Freedom of opinion and expression is a central tenet in international human rights law. At its first session in 1946, the General Assembly described freedom of opinion and expression as "a fundamental human right and the touchstone of all freedoms to which the United Nations is consecrated." The United Nations Conference on Freedom of Information which followed in 1948 produced Article 19 of the Universal Declaration. This section broadly provides: "Everyone has the right to freedom of opinion and expression; this right includes freedom to hold opinions without interference and to seek, receive and impart information and ideas through any media and regardless of frontiers."

Freedom of expression is critical in medicine and health care. Research requires that investigators and participants freely exchange information. Effective education of health care professionals, individuals, and communities depends upon the free flow of accurate scientific and medical information. But freedom of expression in the health care context implies more than the absence of government censorship. The International Bill of Human Rights recognizes the right of all persons "to share in scientific advancement and its benefits" (Universal Declaration, Art. 27.1; similar in Covenant on Economic, Social and Cultural Rights, Art. 15.1[a], [b]). This implies a state obligation to make certain that its population will receive evidence of scientific advances and will share in benefits that may accrue from them. For example, the government might promptly disseminate public health data to all health care practitioners, or provide immunizations to individuals, communities, or nations that could not otherwise obtain them.

Protecting free expression and promoting fair distribution of new scientific and technological advances have profound implications for HIV/AIDS prevention efforts (United Nations [UNAIDS], 1995e). Governments may neither restrict nor criminalize an individual's distribution of information on safe sexual or needle-sharing behaviors. Freedom of expression constitutes a "negative" right; it provides "freedom from" government limits on the imparting or receiving of information.

On the other hand, the right to receive information may be viewed as a "positive" right. Governments are obligated to inform the public about risky behaviors through HIV education and counseling programs and state-developed or sponsored communication networks. Such affirmative steps enable individuals to seek and receive health information vital to their well-being.

Freedom from arbitrary arrest, detention, or exile

Article 9 of the Universal Declaration of Human Rights proclaims: "No one shall be subjected to arbitrary arrest, detention or exile." A similar provision appears in Article

9, paragraph 1, of the International Covenant on Civil and Political Rights: "Everyone has the right to liberty and security of person. No one shall be subjected to arbitrary arrest or detention. No one shall be deprived of his liberty except on such grounds and in accordance with such procedures as are established by law."

Liberty. The right to be free from arbitrary arrest, detention, or exile in the UDHR and ICCPR springs from the right of liberty and security of person. Liberty may be defined as freedom from restraint unless justly imposed by law. The right to liberty does not guarantee immunity from reasonable limitations imposed for the community's interests.

Deprivations of liberty must be "prescribed by law" and cannot be "arbitrary." A restriction is "prescribed by law" if it is born of democratic processes. Such laws, moreover, must be construed within the purpose and spirit of the International Bill of Rights (United Nations, 1990). "Arbitrary" deprivations of liberty are oppressive governmental acts, including capricious arrest, detention, or exile. The word "arbitrary" is intended to encompass both "illegal" and "unjust" acts (United Nations, 1990).

A community may restrict an individual's liberty through a broad array of health policies and institutions. Liberty is diminished, for example, by isolation, quarantine, and civil commitment. Similarly, criminal penalties (e.g., imprisonment, house arrest, or probation against persons with HIV/AIDS) also impinge on the right to liberty.

Natural Justice. The European concept of natural justice, referred to as due process or procedural fairness in some common-law systems, is exercised when a fair and independent hearing is held before a person is deprived of liberty. The government must inform persons why they are being detained and must hold a hearing before an independent court or tribunal prior to detention (or within a reasonable time thereafter). Moreover, the hearing must be before a court that is judicial in character to ensure adequate procedural protections and to safeguard fundamental freedoms, that operates independently of the executive and other parties to the case, and that renders binding decisions (United Nations, 1991a; *X. v. United Kingdom*, 1981; *Van der Leer v. The Netherlands*, 1990).

Within the health context, governments must grant individuals a fair hearing before depriving them of liberty. Thus, before implementing decisions to isolate, quarantine, civilly commit, or compulsorily treat persons, the state must follow a fair procedure which affords the person the opportunity to present relevant evidence and arguments.

Freedom of movement

Freedom of movement subsumes various types of travel, both intra- and interstate. The Universal Declaration of Human Rights claims: "Everyone has the right to freedom of movement and residence within the borders of each State. Everyone has the right to leave any country, including his own, and to return to his country" (Art. 13). The International Covenant of Civil and Political Rights states:

Everyone lawfully within the territory of a State shall, within that territory, have the right to liberty of movement and freedom to choose his residence. Everyone shall be free to leave any country, including his own. . . . No one shall be arbitrarily deprived of the right to enter his own country (Art. 12).

The International Bill of Human Rights does not recognize an absolute right to travel or to immigrate to another country. However, Article 14 of the Universal Declaration guarantees a near-absolute right to seek asylum: "Everyone has the right to seek and to enjoy in other countries asylum from persecution."

The WHO has spearheaded modern efforts to prevent unjustified travel restrictions. The International Health Regulations, issued by the World Health Assembly, designate the one document of health status that can properly be required for international travel: a valid certificate of vaccination against yellow fever (World Health Organization, 1992d). Regarding HIV infection, the World Health Organization has stated that "no country bound by the Regulations may refuse entry into its territory to a person who fails to provide a medical certificate stating that he or she is not carrying the AIDS virus" (International Health Regulations, 1985). Unfortunately, the Regulations have been widely disregarded. Many countries have restricted entry by persons known or suspected to have HIV or AIDS (see Chapter 4: Travel and Immigration Restrictions).

The right to marry and found a family

Article 16 of the Universal Declaration of Human Rights addresses rights relating to the family:

1. Men and women of full age, without any limitation due to race, nationality or religion, have the right to marry and to found a family. They are entitled to equal rights as to marriage, during marriage and at its dissolution. 2. Marriage shall be entered into only with the free and full consent of the intending spouses. 3. The family is the natural and fundamental group unit of society and is entitled to protection by society and the State.

The International Covenant of Civil and Political Rights (ICCPR) also contains a similar right to marry following free and full consent and to found a family. The ICCPR also recognizes the family as the fundamental group unit of society and urges States to offer the family "the widest possible protection and assistance" (Art. 10). Furthermore, the ICCPR demands that States "take appropriate steps to ensure equality of rights and responsibilities of spouses as to marriage, during marriage and at its dissolution. In the case of dissolution, provision shall be made for the necessary protection of any children" (Art. 23). The International Covenant of Economic, Social and Cultural Rights requires the full and free consent of both parties to a marriage.

The Right to Marry. Countries should have a duty to sponsor effective programs to prevent HIV infection within marriage. One approach is to educate, counsel, and test couples voluntarily both before and after marriage. Countries might also integrate HIV prevention activities into child/maternal health and family-planning programs.

Premarital education, counseling, and/or testing have long been part of sexually transmitted infection (STI) and rubella control programs. Such policies do not violate the right to marry, since the infected person may marry after she, for instance, obtains STI treatment or her unexposed partner is immunized against rubella. These policies may, however, impinge upon the right to marry by imposing delays or expense, or by divulging intimate information to a prospective spouse. In most cases, though, the burden is neither unduly invasive nor long-lasting, and is outweighed by a compelling public health purpose.

Many jurisdictions have devised premarital HIV-prevention policies based on STI programs (Thomas, 1987). These programs may minimally burden human rights if the testing is voluntary and, with informed consent, the couple is allowed to marry.

Premarital screening for STIs or HIV has generally been abandoned for two reasons. First, mass screening for HIV can be quite expensive and may detect few cases, particularly in areas with a low prevalence (Field, 1990; Cleary, Barry, et al., 1987). Second, premarital screening may be only marginally effective in preventing HIV infection. Many couples engage in sexual intercourse before marriage; HIV infection may already have been transmitted. Even if one partner is HIV-negative, she may not possess the power within her culture to withdraw from a proposed marriage. Policymakers must ask whether the resources expended for premarital screening could be better utilized for other, more cost-effective HIV prevention programs.

If structured coercively, premarital screening programs may mandate testing without consent or deny a marriage license if one or both partners test positive. Compulsory premarital screening, even if it does not lead to a ban on marriage, might paradoxically discourage people from applying for marriage licenses. In one jurisdiction, the number of marriage licenses issued dropped sharply after the state instituted a program of compulsory premarital screening (Illinois Department of Public Health, 1989).

An outright ban on marriage for HIV-infected persons would directly violate the right to marry as specified in the UDHR, the ICCPR, and the ICESCR. Moreover, public health grounds cannot adequately justify such a policy; banning marriage will not prevent the spread of HIV since unmarried people can still engage in practices that transmit the virus. Furthermore, married or not, persons can use protective measures to prevent transmission.

Whether any premarital testing program may be justified on public health grounds depends on a number of factors, including the voluntariness of the program, the inclusion of adequate pre- and post-test counseling, the seroprevalence in the population, and the resources available for HIV control programs. Testing programs that are mandatory, impose bans on marriage, or threaten the right to privacy of potential spouses by compelling disclosure to persons other than the potential marriage partners may negatively impact AIDS prevention efforts. Any coercive measure may lead people to distrust public health authorities or discourage testing. Since prevention requires long-lasting, voluntary behavior change, measures that facilitate cooperation and education are likely to be more effective than those that instill fear or distrust (World Health Organization, 1987c). In contrast, a premarital program that promotes counseling all potential spouses about the risks of HIV infection and the means to avoid it, and voluntarily tests following informed consent, can be an integral part of a wider AIDS prevention program. The knowledge that such programs impart may effect behavior changes which can protect both partners from HIV infection.

The Right to Found a Family. The right of HIV-infected persons to found a family poses vexing ethical issues. Here, the parental right to have children may conflict with the responsibility to protect children from harm. Reproductive rights of women and men are significant human rights. A constellation of human entitlements supports the interrelated rights to engage in sexual relationships, to procreate, and to found a family (Cook, 1992, 1993). All persons possess the rights to autonomy and freedom of association, which entitle them to choose their relations and decide for themselves the benefits and risks of procreation. People are, moreover, entitled to privacy in their relationships. In making judgments about reproduction and the welfare of future offspring, it is the woman (in consultation with her partner) who is best positioned to decide about her bodily integrity and the child's welfare.

Governmental interference (e.g., prohibiting or restricting the right of HIV-infected women or men from having children) not only infringes on the person's right to found a family but may also affect future generations of whole communities (often disfavored minorities who may bear a disproportionate burden of HIV). Throughout history, governments have made infamous decisions to sterilize or otherwise limit the reproductive choices of vulnerable citizens who were mentally retarded or had genetic or infectious diseases that could be transmitted perinatally. Government-imposed decisions to limit reproductive choices are often imbued with value judgments suggesting that certain prospective parents are incapable of evaluating the risks and benefits of having children, and that children with disabilities are unable to live full and purposeful lives.

Health agencies do, however, have a duty to reduce perinatal transmission of HIV. Thus, health officials must adequately inform women and men of reproductive age about the risks of vertical transmission and arm them with the knowledge and means to lower those risks. The meaning and importance of childbearing and the significance of the risk to offspring will be evaluated differently by public health authorities and by women and men in different countries, cultures, and economic positions. The risk of perinatal HIV transmission continues to be estimated at twenty-five to thirty-five percent. Where zidovudine (AZT) is available (e.g., in more developed countries), its use can sharply reduce the risk of vertical transmission (Centers for Disease Control, 1994). Current research explores the efficacy and feasibility of less costly means of prevention, including short courses of zidovudine and obstetrical practices such as cleansing of the birth canal (vaginal lavage) (Bryson, 1996). Current data indicate that even without intervention, up to three-quarters (or higher) of babies born to HIV-infected mothers do *not* become infected with HIV. Moreover, HIV infection is not the only dangerous condition, infectious or hereditary, with which a child can be born. In societies where a woman's status, self-worth, and possibly even survival in marriage depend upon her fertility, many women will be willing to risk giving birth to an infected child (Levine, Dubler, 1990). Women who are not HIV-infected—but who are married to men who are either infected or at high risk of infection—may continue to have unprotected sexual intercourse because they want, or feel pressured to have, children (United Nations, 1992).

Women's groups in Africa and elsewhere have argued that as long as childbearing is so highly valued, the promotion of condoms or other "safer sex" practices will have a limited impact on HIV transmission between spouses or potential spouses. These groups have called for research to develop practical forms of virucides (substances capable of killing HIV) which do not simultaneously prevent conception (Elias, Heise, 1993; Williams, 1992, personal communication). Despite a woman's wishes to use a barrier method of contraception that protects against HIV transmission, she may be prevented from doing so by her partner or by the unavailability of contraceptives.

Perhaps a more difficult matter is whether an HIV-infected man possesses the right to found a family. With the current state of contraceptives and viricidal technology, any efforts by an HIV-infected man to procreate poses a risk of infection to both his partner and any potential offspring. In societies that value large families, men as well as women, regardless of their HIV status, may feel pressured to have children.

Adoption remains a relatively safe way for men and women with HIV infection to found a family. Some jurisdictions have considered testing adoptive parents for HIV. Since HIV infection is not spread through casual contact, HIV infection of a parent would constitute a contraindication to adoption only in that the parent might not live long enough to raise the child to majority. Proposals for testing adoptive parents for HIV should be evaluated in the context of other existing health requirements, the availability of resources, and the need for adoptive parents. Unfortunately, the HIV/AIDS pandemic is leaving many orphans in the hardest-hit geographic areas—an estimated 5.5 million in Africa alone by the year 2000 (Preble, 1990). To exclude HIV-infected parents from adopting would negatively impact HIV prevention and control efforts if doing so encourages these parents to have biological children, increases discrimination or stigmatization of those with HIV, consumes scarce resources, or significantly reduces the pool of potential adoptive parents.

The Requirement of Free and Full Consent of Both Parties to a Marriage. Women who are coerced or sold into marriage do not make an autonomous choice. Once married, they are likely to continue to have little autonomy. Economic and social dependence on their husbands may leave them unable to protect themselves from exposure to HIV by insisting that their husbands use condoms. Women, who, after being widowed, are "inherited" or expected to wed their husband's relative—and young girls who are given, exchanged, or sold into marriage—are unlikely to protect themselves in marriage (see 9, below).

The requirement that marriage only be entered into with the free and full consent of both parties offers protection from such abuses. Nonetheless, it is insufficient; even though a woman knows she may risk her health, she may consent to a marriage if she sees it as the only socially acceptable alternative. In many societies, consent of both parties that is truly "full and free" will require an improved status for women, including economic independence and increased authority and responsibility in decision-making within marriage (Hausermann, Danziger, 1991).

Equal Rights and Responsibilities Within Marriage and upon Dissolution. National laws and enforcement standards often leave a gaping discrepancy between the rights of women as enunciated in international legal texts and the reality of women's lives.

> In many cases, national laws contravene international human rights norms by, for instance, denying women the right to own property, and acquire mortgages and other forms of financial credit. They frequently limit the women's rights within marriage and, on separation or divorce, deny women equal custodial rights to their children (Hausermann, Danziger, 1991).

In many societies women possess little decision-making power inside marriage and lack protection of property or economic support upon dissolution of the marriage. Laws or social practices which reinforce women's economic dependency on men increase women's vulnerability in many ways. Young women often have no real alternative to marriage, making them unable to decline a proposed husband, even one who has HIV infection or practices high-risk behaviors. Once married, women often are not able to influence their husbands' extramarital sexual behavior or to protect themselves from unsafe sex. They may be sexually assaulted or threatened with abandonment if they refuse unprotected sex. Women who lose their spouse through death or divorce often have no means, other than prostitution, to support themselves and their children.

Freedom from slavery and similar practices

The Universal Declaration of Human Rights (Art. 4) and the International Covenant on Civil and Political Rights (Art. 8) both state: "No one shall be held in slavery or servitude; slavery and the slave trade shall be prohibited." After more than a century of intensive effort, the international movement succeeded in implementing this ban.

The League of Nations approved the International Slavery Convention in 1926. In 1953, the United Nations incorporated the League of Nations' powers outlined in the 1926 Convention. The Convention defined slavery as "the status or condition of a person over whom any or all of the powers attaching to the right of ownership are exercised." The slave trade included:

> all acts involved in the capture, acquisition or disposal of a person with intent to reduce him to slavery; all acts involved in the acquisition of a slave with a view to selling or exchanging him; all acts of disposal by sale or exchange of a slave acquired with a view to being sold or exchanged, and, in general, every act of trade or transport in slaves (International Slavery Convention, 1926).

Since 1953, the international community has adopted conventions concerning practices that resemble slavery but do not fit within the 1926 definition. For example, in 1956, the Supplementary Convention on the Abolition of Slavery, the Slave Trade, and Institutions and Practices Similar to Slavery was adopted. This document calls upon member countries to end practices including debt bondage; serfdom; the sale, purchase, exchange, or inheritance of a woman for marriage or upon the death of her husband; and the transferal of a child under age eighteen to exploit the child's labor.

Suppression of Traffic for Commercial Sex Work.

International treaties aimed at suppressing traffic in persons for prostitution similarly predated the League of Nations and the United Nations (United Nations, 1984, pp. 48–49). In 1950, the United Nations consolidated these treaties in its Convention for the Suppression of the Traffic in Persons and of the Exploitation of the Prostitution of Others. This Convention obligates parties to punish persons who recruit or procure prostitutes; keep, manage, or finance brothels; or knowingly rent a building for that purpose. The United Nations, however, did little to apply these provisions. Subsequently, the Commission on the Status of Women, the Economic and Social Council, and international conferences have sought to convince countries that commercial sex work is a serious offense against women and children's dignity and to identify socioeconomic conditions that precipitate it. In 1983, the report of the Special Rapporteur, Jean Fernand-Laurent, led the General Assembly to conclude that commercial sex work and the accompanying evil of traffic in persons for the purpose of prostitution were incompatible with human dignity and worth and endangered the welfare of the individual, family, and community.

For several reasons, the persistence of slavery-like practices is relevant to the HIV/AIDS context. First, people who are forced into marriage, prostitution, or other labor suffer losses in autonomy that disempower them from safeguarding their health. For example, women who are coerced or sold into marriage often have no realistic alternative for economic independence. Since they face destitution or worse if the marriage ends, they are poorly positioned to demand that their partner use a condom, even if they know or suspect he is infected with HIV (see The Right to Marry and Found a Family, earlier). Women who are "inherited" by a family member following a husband's death may unwillingly be exposed to a source of HIV infection or may themselves expose another family member to HIV. Women or men who are transported from developing countries to work in industrialized countries may become virtual captives of their employers. They may not be able to refuse unwanted sexual advances for fear of physical abuse or deprivation. Women or children who are sold into prostitution usually cannot choose their customers or insist upon condom use. Moreover, husbands, brothel owners, or employers frequently deny women and children access to information, education, and the means to protect themselves from HIV infection.

HIV/AIDS has a second, somewhat paradoxical impact on the business of commercial sex work. In areas where people perceive the risk of HIV infection to be high, many customers opt for young children, believing them less likely to be HIV-infected. As the demand for young sex workers increases, brothel keepers expand their "resource pools." They do so by coercing or bribing parents in foreign countries and in economically depressed regions to sell their children (knowingly or unknowingly) to houses of prostitution (United Nations, 1992). Young sex workers who become HIV-infected find themselves further punished by legal systems which should have protected them in the first place. They may face multiple legal sanctions: punishment for breach of prostitution or immigration laws and state coercion or discrimination under HIV/AIDS laws, policies, or practices (United Nations, 1992a).

Finally, commercial sex work raises human rights concerns even absent the forced procurement or sale of women and children. The international community has long recognized that poverty, lack of economic alternatives, and the low social status of women undergird the problem of commercial sex work. During the last decade, worsening economic conditions in many countries, civil and international conflicts leading to many displaced persons, as well as the increasing "feminization of poverty" that has accompanied the AIDS pandemic have led many women, girls, and boys into prostitution as a matter of economic survival. Thus, improving women's social and economic status is crucial to reducing the exploitation of women through prostitution and to decreasing their risk of HIV infection (United Nations, 1989f). Women's greater economic stability would benefit both themselves and their children. Consequently, fewer children themselves might be driven to commercial sex work. Sex workers who are homosexuals, transsexuals, or transvestites are often further discriminated against and are particularly vulnerable to exploitation and abuse. Measures that protect sexual minorities from discrimination in employment, housing, and education could reduce their exploitation.

Economic, Social, and Cultural Rights

The HIV/AIDS pandemic underscores the problems of inadequate resources, unequal development, social injustice, and pervasive discrimination. Since the ICESCR was drafted, these obstacles have impeded the full realization of economic, social, and cultural rights, including the right to health (United Nations, 1984, pp. 92–93). The countries that incur the greatest costs of the HIV/AIDS pandemic are among the poorest. The World Health Organization estimates that nearly ninety percent of the HIV infections and AIDS cases of the 1990s are occurring in developing countries. A significant investment of resources is sorely needed to help these countries both combat AIDS and narrow the gulf between developed and developing countries' realization of economic, social, and cultural rights.

The right to health

The notion that human beings are entitled to health is derived from numerous international documents (Jamar, 1994; Leary, 1994; Harvard Law School Human Rights Program, 1995). The preamble of the World Health Organization's Constitution (1946), states: "The enjoyment of the highest attainable standard of health is one of the fundamental rights of every human being without distinction of race, religion, political belief, economic or social conditions." The UN Charter itself dedicates the United Nations to promoting solutions for international health problems (Art. 55). The UDHR proclaims a right to "a standard of living adequate for the health and well-being of individuals and their families" (Art. 25). The Convention of the Rights of the Child recognizes the right of children to the enjoyment of the "highest attainable standard of health" (Art. 24[1]).

The ICESCR recognizes "the right of everyone to the highest attainable standard of physical and mental health." Party states agree to take steps to fully realize this right, including those necessary for:

> (a) The provision for the reduction of the stillbirth-rate and of infant mortality and for the healthy development of the child; (b) The improvement of all aspects of environmental and industrial hygiene; (c) The prevention, treatment and control of epidemic, endemic, occupational and other diseases; (d) The creation of conditions which would assure to all medical service and medical attention in the event of sickness (Art. 12).

The WHO and UNICEF Declaration of Alma Ata (1978) reaffirms that:

> health, which is a state of complete physical, mental and social well-being, and not merely the absence of disease or infirmity, is a fundamental human right and that the attainment of the highest possible level of health is a most important world-wide social goal whose realization requires the action of many other social and economic sectors in addition to the health sector.

In 1981, The World Health Assembly unanimously adopted the Global Strategy for Health for All by the Year 2000 (United Nations, 1984, p. 93). Several regional human rights documents, as well as national constitutions, also recognize a right to health (African Charter on Human and Peoples' Rights, Art. 16; American Declaration of the Rights and Duties of Man, Art. 11; European Social Charter, Art. 11; Fuenzalida-Puelma, Connor, 1989).

Various international documents emphasize the role of nondiscrimination in promoting and protecting the right to health. The Convention on the Elimination of All Forms of Discrimination Against Women, for example, pledges states to take all appropriate steps to eliminate discrimination against women in health care and to ensure women access to appropriate services in connection with childbearing (Art. 12). Similarly, the Convention on the Elimination of All Forms of Racial Discrimination proscribes racial discrimination in the enjoyment of the right to health (Art. 5[e][iv]).

The conceptualization of health as a human right, and not simply a moral claim, suggests that states possess binding obligations to respect, defend, and promote that entitlement. Considerable disagreement, however, exists as to whether "health" is a meaningful, identifiable, operational, and enforceable right, or whether it is merely aspirational. A right to health that is too broadly defined lacks clear content and is less likely to have a meaningful impact. For example, if health is, in the World Health Organization's words, truly "a state of complete physical, mental and social well-being," then it can never be achieved. Even if this definition were construed as a reasonable, as opposed to an absolute, standard (Leary, 1994), it remains difficult to implement and is unlikely to be justiciable.

The international community (United Nations, 1993a) and legal scholars (Jamar, 1994) have begun to craft a definition of the right to health that clarifies state obligations, identifies violations, and establishes criteria and procedures for enforcement. Here, we offer suggestions for a workable definition, but we recognize that considerable development is needed.

The Institute of Medicine (1988, p. 19) proposes a thoughtful definition of public health:

> Public health is what we, as a society, do collectively to assure the conditions for people to be healthy. This requires that continuing and emerging threats to the health of the public be successfully countered. These threats include immediate crises, such as the AIDS epidemic; enduring problems, such as injuries and chronic illness; and growing challenges, such as the aging of our population and the toxic by-products of a modern economy, transmitted through air, water, soil, or food. These and many other problems raise in common the need to protect the nation's health through effective, organized, and sustained efforts led by the public sector.

Building on this definition, the right to health may be defined as "The duty of the state, within the limits of its available resources, to ensure the conditions necessary for the health of individuals and populations." This definition achieves several purposes, but also harbors a number of weaknesses. Most importantly, the definition places explicit obligations on the state and recognizes that a claim requires a correlating duty. By acknowledging that states possess varying capabilities, this definition also requires a state to act only within the limits of its resources to secure the right to health. The definition does not impose an absolute standard of physical and mental health. Health is the result of many factors outside of government's control, such as genetics, behavior, overpopulation, and climate; to designate the state as the guarantor of a particular level of physical and mental health is unrealistic and may divert attention from individual responsibility for a person's own health. However, the state does possess the power to ensure the conditions under which people can be healthy. Governments can do a great deal to improve the health of individuals and populations, including providing decent sanitation, hygiene, clean air, clean water, nutrition, clothing, housing, medical care, disease surveillance and control, vaccinations, and health education and promotion. Government obligations, then, go beyond the provision of discrete medical services (Chapman, 1993) to the assurance of a broad array of services that are necessary for populations to maintain health. Minimally, the state would have a responsibility, within the limits of its available resources, to intervene to prevent or reduce serious threats to the health of individuals or populations. The definition's principal disadvantage is that it does not ensure a minimal standard of health and allows differential responses to health threats based on the available economic resources.

Vast scholarship and litigation in national and international fora were required to define and enforce civil and political rights. Economic and social rights, notably the right to health, require the same sustained attention.

The right to education

The International Bill of Human Rights guarantees all persons the right to an education (UDHR, Art. 26; ICESCR, Art. 13.14). Pursuant to the UDHR and ICESCR, states agree that education should develop human dignity and personality. The right to education encompasses information and counseling on health risks, disease prevention, and practical forms of self-protection.

The rights to both education and health are integrally interconnected; one cannot be achieved without the other. In the absence of a vaccine or cure for HIV/AIDS, education remains the single most important method of disease prevention. The right to education is not simply the unemcumbered right to disseminate relevant information; it necessitates careful research and planning to devise education strategies that effectively reduce health risks. Behavioral research suggests several methods for effective AIDS education (Institute of Medicine, 1994). The population needs accurate information about behaviors that increase the risk of transmission. Clear, comprehensible information that is suitable to local language, literacy levels, and culture about the risks of sexual, needle-borne, and perinatal transmission is indispensable to education efforts. The resources devoted to education, and the messages used, will vary with the population. Furthermore, education must specifically target groups that are particularly vulnerable or at increased risk of infection.

Since effective HIV/AIDS education seeks to change many intimate and ingrained behaviors, such as sex and drug use, it often conflicts with equally entrenched social or religious norms. Governments, health care providers, or other organizations attempting to change people's behaviors must be responsive to the needs and sensitivities of the community. Focused education of the community on the pressing public health need for targeted, accurate, and complete HIV/AIDS prevention education is a vital first step in overcoming community resistance to efforts to elicit behavior change.

Sound education must inform the population how to reduce risk. Clear instructions regarding safer sex, drug injection, and reproductive choices enable individuals to protect themselves and their partners from HIV/AIDS. Social scientists have long understood that even where populations are well informed about health risks, behavior does not change unless individuals acquire the means to protect themselves. Knowledge alone will not reduce the risk of HIV transmission; people also need access to condoms or sterile injection equipment to reduce episodes of unprotected sex or needle sharing. Even where the means are available, individuals may further need to learn new techniques or skills. For example, a woman who is trapped, culturally and economically, in a relationship may need to be empowered before she can insist that her partner wear a condom. Similarly, a commercial sex worker may need more than condoms to reduce her occupational risk of infection. The right to education, then, is connected to health in a fundamental way, and may require a range of strategies—including full and culturally appropriate information, interventions targeted to vulnerable groups, and the means, skill, and power necessary to change behavior—to achieve success.

The right to an adequate standard of living, including food and shelter

"Everyone has the right to a standard of living adequate for the health and well-being of himself and his family, including food, clothing, housing and medical care" (UDHR, Art. 25). The ICESCR also calls upon States to recognize the fundamental right of all persons to be free from hunger (Art. 11). Promotion of this right reduces people's vulnerability to a myriad of health risks, including HIV infection.

The right to an adequate standard of living, like the right to education, is integral to the right to health. Food, clothing, housing, and health care are all requisites for human health. Persons who lack these necessities face direct and indirect health threats. Malnutrition, exposure to extreme weather conditions (e.g., cold, heat, or flooding), and lack of basic health care (e.g., family planning, pre- and postnatal care, immunizations, antibiotics, and oral rehydration) produce preventable morbidity and mortality. Similarly, persons who lack adequate food, housing, and health care are at increased risk of exposure to disease. For example, homeless persons are more likely to encounter malaria-carrying mosquitos, and those who are malnourished are more likely to progress from tuberculosis infection to active disease. The subsequent risks affect not only those persons without an adequate standard of living but the rest of the population as well.

An inadequate standard of living is particularly threatening to persons with immuno-compromising conditions, such as HIV. A person with AIDS who lacks decent shelter, clothing, food, and health care is significantly more likely to develop pernicious and fulminating opportunistic infections than those with adequate access to these services.

The right to share in the benefits of scientific and technological progress

Everyone possesses the right to share in the benefits of scientific advancements and their technological applications (ICESCR, Art. 15; UDHR, Art. 27). The United Nations General Assembly has requested member states to "promote access of all peoples to appropriate preventive, diagnostic, and therapeutic technologies and pharmaceuticals, and to help make these technologies and pharmaceuticals available at an affordable cost" (United Nations, 1989a).

The right to share in the benefits of scientific progress has particular import in the HIV/AIDS pandemic. Many technologies have already been developed to prevent, care for, and treat HIV/AIDS; many more technologies are needed. Cost-effective innovations—such as HIV testing (e.g., to screen the blood supply), infection control measures in health care settings (e.g., gloves and sterile medical instruments), antiviral medications and treatments for opportunistic infections, strategies to reduce the biological or behavioral risks of transmission, and eventually even vaccinations and cures—must be shared globally. As science develops new technologies to combat HIV/AIDS, the need to ensure availability in all countries—poorer, as well as richer—becomes more pressing (Parker, 1996).

The right to development

Perhaps the most basic issue underlying the realization of all economic, social, and cultural rights is the right to development. In 1986, the United Nations General Assembly defined development as "a comprehensive economic, social, cultural and political process, that aims at the constant improvement of the well-being of the entire population and of all individuals on the basis of their active, free and meaningful participation in development and in the fair distribution of benefits resulting therefrom" (United Nations, 1986). The United Nations World Conference on Human Rights reaffirmed the right of development as "universal and inalienable . . . and an integral part of fundamental human rights" (Vienna Declaration and Programme of Action, 1993).

At an international consultation sponsored by the United Nations, experts proposed measures by which to realize the right to development. The criteria included conditions of life (food, shelter, housing, health, education, personal freedom, and security), conditions of work, and equality of access to resources and participation. Members of the Consultation suggested that donor countries, agencies, and developing countries too often define "development" narrowly to refer only to economic growth; in their view, social justice deserves attention as well. Consultation members called upon parties to define development more broadly and to regard human rights as a cornerstone to future efforts (United Nations, 1991b).

The HIV/AIDS pandemic is an economic, social, and cultural concern as well as a public health problem. Consequently, all economic, social, and cultural rights—including the right to education, an adequate standard of living, the benefits of scientific progress, and development—are fundamental to ensuring the conditions in which people can be healthy.

CHALLENGES IN THE EVOLUTION OF HUMAN RIGHTS DOCTRINE

International human rights doctrine has evolved subject to certain competing interests. These tensions include, for example, the sovereignty of the state versus the right of the individual as a subject of international law, and the significance of claims of the individual versus those of the community or population. Many disagreements about whether and how to apply or enforce human rights represent theoretical disagreements about the fundamental character of human rights. Claims of national sovereignty, cultural differences in rights' recognition or interpretation, distinctions between positive and negative rights, and conflicts over group versus individual rights go to the heart of human rights theory. To offer a sense of the rich complexity of international human rights doctrine, the following section examines three threshold issues encountered during its evolution. These examples are merely illustrative of this growing and robust body of law.

Debate has alternately hindered and advanced the development of international human rights law, and continues to inform, both positively and negatively, the international community's interpretation and application of that law. The human rights framework is dynamic. As such, it presents abundant possibilities for growth and flexibility within the system and constitutes an important approach to advancing and protecting rights and promoting health during the HIV/AIDS pandemic.

What Is a Right Without a Remedy? Problems with Enforcement, Justiciability, and Standard-Setting

The tension between individual rights and permissible limitations: when does the exception become the rule?

As previously noted, few rights are absolute. Although human rights instruments prohibit the state from infringing upon particular individual rights, so, too, do they permit the state to limit or suspend certain rights under specific circumstances.

The instruments of the International Bill of Human Rights prescribe the conditions under which states may impinge upon these rights. Each instrument stipulates that it may not "be interpreted as implying for any State, group or person any right to engage in any activity or perform any act aimed at the destruction of any of the rights and freedoms recognized herein" (UDHR, Art. 30; ICCPR and ICESCR, Art. 5.1). The Covenants specify that their provisions may not be construed to limit the rights recognized to a greater extent than provided for in the instrument itself (ICCPR and ICESCR, Art. 5.1). Nor may they be interpreted to restrict a country's other fundamental human rights granted by law or custom on the pretext that the Covenant either does not recognize the right or provides a lesser protection (ICCPR and ICESCR, Art. 5.2).

On the other hand, the instruments expressly permit states to implement measures, under certain circumstances, that limit or suspend particular rights. Article 4 of the ICCPR declares that states may deviate from their Covenant (1) during an officially proclaimed period of "public emergency which threatens the life of the nation"; (2) to the "extent strictly required by the exigencies of the situation"; and (3) insofar as such derogation measures are not applied in a discriminatory manner. Certain rights may not be diminished under the ICCPR: the rights to life; to be recognized as a person; and to freedom of thought, conscience, and religion; the prohibition against torture and cruel or inhuman treatment; slavery; ex post facto offenses; and imprisonment for inability to fulfill a contractual obligation. Other articles of the ICCPR expressly allow limitations of protected rights, usually where prescribed by law and necessary to protect a substantial social goal, such as public order (Art. 12, 14, 18, 19, 22), national security (Art. 12, 13, 14, 19, 21, 22), public safety (Art. 18, 21, 22), or protection of the rights of others (Art. 12, 18, 19, 21, 22). The protection of public health or morals is a permissible justification for limiting rights recognized in Articles 12, 14, 18, 19, 21, and 22.

Article 4 of the ICESCR contains a general provision which allows restriction of recognized rights where provided for by law, "compatible with the nature of these rights," and protective of "the general welfare in a democratic society." Trade union rights (Art. 8) are also subject to certain specific limitations.

Given the latitude of the limitations enunciated in the instruments, not to mention the frequency of state failure to honor human rights obligations generally, the exceptions may seem to subsume the very protections to be enforced. The suspension or restriction of rights under states of emergency is particularly problematic (Oraá, 1992). A strong correlation exists between states of emergency and grave human rights violations (International Commission of Jurists, 1983). Many purported exigencies have masked the unjustified infringement of individual rights.

To respond to the human rights restrictions, one must first examine their interpretation, application, and enforcement (Diemer, 1986). Under the ICCPR, the state possesses the authority to decide when conditions "threaten the life of the nation" or to suggest alternative criteria upon which to limit or suspend an otherwise protected right. The state determinations trigger the Convention's compliance mechanisms, which then assess whether the state's conclusion is factually and legally supported. The HRC may offer general comments through its usual reporting function or exercise its duty to scrutinize a particular case submitted under the Optional Protocol. The HRC begins by interpreting the text, perhaps guided by reference to additional standards and the considerable corpus of international jurisprudence that has developed around this issue.

Standards have been promulgated to delineate circumstances of permissible derogation. For example, a group of international law experts drafted the Siracusa Principles on the Limitation and Derogation Provisions in the ICCPR in an effort to clarify and construe those clauses (Siracusa Principles, 1984). In the context of health-related rights, for example, the Siracusa Principles allow that "[p]ublic health may be invoked as a ground for limiting certain rights in order to allow the state to take measures dealing with a serious threat to the health of the population" or of individuals. Such measures must be "specifically aimed at preventing disease or injury or providing care for the sick and injured." WHO's international health regulations are to serve as a reference (Siracusa Principles, 1984, pp. 25, 26). The Limburg Principles on the Implementation of the ICESCR, inter alia, address the limitations clauses of that instrument.

Any justification for limiting individual rights should signal the need to strictly scrutinize the justification and circumstances. Allowing states to limit individual rights was not intended to allow derogation at will. The Covenants designate the circumstances under which restriction of rights is permitted; these circumstances must be closely construed and vigorously enforced, particularly when the justifications involve public health emergencies. Compulsory measures, invoked to combat the spread of disease, may create a paradox. Measures such as compulsory testing, isolation, and quarantine may help prevent the transmission of certain airborne diseases (e.g., tuberculosis), but can be counterproductive in containing other diseases (e.g., HIV/AIDS). Specifically, by restricting the autonomy, privacy, or liberty of persons at risk of HIV, the government may alienate and antagonize those whom it most seeks to align with health care and public health professionals. As a result, emergency efforts may actually thwart public health goals.

The problem of justiciability and standard-setting for economic, social, and cultural rights

Many economic, social, and cultural rights are by their nature difficult to define. In addition, international documents allow that countries may gradually implement these rights, further confounding efforts to determine what constitutes a violation and the standard by which to measure a country's progress. Due to the inherent problems of definition, measurement, monitoring, and enforcement, some commentators have questioned the usefulness or validity of acknowledging economic, social, and cultural rights (*The Economist*, 1993).

For example, the ICESCR treats the right to health (Art. 12) generally rather than specifically. The right to health itself is not defined. Moreover, although Article 12 calls for affirmative acts (e.g., measures to reduce the stillbirth rate and infant mortality or measures to prevent, treat, and control various forms of disease), no provision designates a minimum standard or denotes a scale of measurement. Similarly, the ICESCR provides that steps be taken toward fully realizing health and improving "all aspects of environmental and industrial hygiene." However, how is the ECOSOC to evaluate compliance? For example, how is "improvement" measured, and how much is needed to constitute a "step"? Article 2 of the ICESCR offers only general guidance, instructing states to initiate efforts "to the maximum of available resources, with a view to achieving progressively the full realization of the rights recognized."

The most apparent solution for applying the ICESCR's rights is to develop more explicit implementation standards. The development and articulation of enhanced standards reflect the dynamic nature of human rights doctrine. The Economic and Social Council, for example, convened a consultation to consider appropriate indicators of achievement in progressively realizing economic, social, and cultural rights (Geneva, 25–29 January 1993). The consultation concluded that whatever indicators are chosen for a particular right or group of rights should be able to detect disparities in the realization of rights, both within and between countries (Committee for Development Planning, 1993; American Association for the Advancement of Science, 1993). Indicators should be particularly sensitive to differences in health status between genders, geographic areas, urban and rural populations, and defined socioeconomic groups.

As previously discussed, international organizations, human rights scholars, and advocates have recently begun to probe the dimensions of the right to health (Committee for Development Planning, 1993; United Nations, 1993a,b; World Health Organization, 1993d; Leary, 1994; Jamar, 1994; also see above, The Right to Health). Scholars and advocates must rigorously consider methods to evaluate and measure the right to health, as well as other economic and social rights. Scholarship and ECOSOC deliberations are at an early stage; with thoughtful appraisal and careful crafting, there is no reason to believe that realistic methods for assessing economic and social rights cannot be devised and implemented on an international level.

That the full scope of economic, social, and cultural rights is still emerging does not, however, detract from the force of these rights as entitlements. As Philip Alston, the chair of the United Nations Economic and Social Council has noted, economic, social, and cultural rights are formally embraced in the West. All western countries except the United States have ratified the ICESCR, and the majority of NGOs have endorsed the validity of these rights. Alston (1993, 1993a) suggests that economic, social, and cultural rights provide important normative standards whose scope, strengths, and weaknesses are just beginning to be explored. He proposes three steps to incorporate fully economic, social, and cultural rights into the corpus of international human rights law: (1) All countries must ratify the ICESCR; (2) all countries must establish the domestic capability to monitor the enjoyment of these rights; and (3) the international community should begin drafting an optional protocol to the ICESCR, creating a complaint and investigation process for alleged violations of these rights.

Problems with enforcement do not vitiate the rights of the individual, but do demonstrate the need to take further steps

Implementation and enforcement of human rights norms challenge those who seek to harmonize human rights and public health. Flagrant and unconscionable human rights abuses continue to occur. For example, although torture constitutes one of the most universally condemned human rights abuses, it continues to be practiced (Human Rights Watch, 1995; Amnesty International, 1993, 1984). The systematic rape of women and slaughter or banishment of ethnic groups in Eastern Europe and Africa demonstrate the intractability of human rights abuses.

As Professor Higgins has noted, challenges do not mean, as some would contend, that "without a remedy, there may not be a right. . . . This approach again looks at things from the perspective of the state, rather than from that of the individual. Problems about delivery leave his right a right nonetheless" (Higgins, 1994). Rather, these challenges indicate that much work remains to clarify, operationalize, and realize the potential of the rights framework.

> As the 20th century draws to a close, human rights in the world are confronted with many serious challenges and threats, including—to mention but a few—war and violence, hunger and poverty, unfair distribution of wealth in the world and within our

societies, aggressive nationalism, intolerance, racism, anti-semitism, xenophobia and religious fanaticism and fundamentalism.

Human rights should not be regarded as a kind of miraculous cure for all the world's ills. It nevertheless seems possible, indeed necessary, for the phenomena just mentioned to be approached from the standpoint of human rights as well. Perhaps their persistence or resurgence is due, amongst other things, to the fact that human rights and the fundamental principles underlying them are being rejected or insufficiently practiced and applied, if indeed at all (Lalumiere, 1993).

When Rights Conflict: Are All Rights Equal?

Negative and positive rights

The status of civil and political rights on the one hand and economic, social, and cultural rights on the other has inspired conflicts and even divisions among the human rights community. In June 1993, at the United Nations Conference on Human Rights in Vienna, contentious debate erupted over whether economic, social, and cultural rights were as pressing as civil and political rights. Similar discussions have occurred at other international meetings such as the International Conference on Population and Development held in Cairo, 5–13 September, 1994 and the Fourth World Conference on Women held in Beijing, 4–15 September, 1995. From a human rights perspective, both sets of rights are equally compelling; both promote the goal of international human rights law: to further the dignity of and respect for all human beings (Leckie, 1990).

Human rights discourse has developed various ways to describe and classify substantive rights. What has not emerged, however, is a uniform practice or meaning for even some common terms. For instance, the terms negative and positive rights are sometimes used, inaccurately, to mean civil and political, as well as economic, social, and cultural rights.

A negative right implies that one has a duty to refrain from doing something to another. In contrast, a positive right suggests that one is obliged to act affirmatively toward another. Some theorists posit that because negative rights require restraint rather than affirmative intervention, the state does not need to expend resources to secure the entitlement. On the other hand, positive rights are assumed to consume resources to implement programs and services necessary to realize the right.

Although offering a neat categorization, this distinction between rights may be misleading. Many civil and political rights, even those designated as "negative" rights, require affirmative state intervention and substantial monetary costs (Sieghart, 1985). The right to a fair trial, for example, requires expenditures to establish and maintain a competent and independent court system and to properly train judges, lawyers, and court personnel. Similarly, the right to participate in free and fair elections requires human and material resources to register voters, set up polling stations, and monitor elections. Conversely, certain economic, social, and cultural rights require little state action or financing. For example, the right to form a trade union requires no government funding and the right of groups to maintain their cultural practices often requires little more than government restraint.

Some persons have invoked the distinction between negative and positive rights to justify a hierarchy of rights. Whether the distinction can be clearly described and maintained, however, may not be the core issue (Lichtenberg, 1982; Shue, 1979, 1980). One might theoretically and validly distinguish between negative and positive rights and still maintain that both are important. Governmental restraint is necessary for individuals to be free of unjustified interference with their liberty interests. Affirmative state action is no less essential to ensure human development and the conditions under which individuals may exercise their freedoms. To facilitate only negative rights creates a climate of "benign neglect." Moreover, rights which protect against governmental interference may be of little interest to persons who lack food, shelter, health care, or work.

Prioritizing competing claims

Human rights law is challenged when competing individuals or groups clash over rights. International human rights law only partially addresses this problem. The UDHR states:

> In the exercise of his rights and freedoms, everyone shall be subject only to such limitations as are determined by law solely for the purpose of securing due recognition and respect for the rights and freedoms of others and of meeting the just requirements of morality, public order and the general welfare in a democratic society (Art. 29).

This provision has been construed as recognizing the need, under certain circumstances, to limit the rights of individuals where they pose a threat to the general welfare. For example, in the public health context, threats to public health may support the need for communicable disease control laws (United Nations, 1990).

Human rights law strives to accomplish a just balancing of rights. Instances exist, however, where achieving such a balance is a formidable challenge. To resolve such conflicts, rights theorists have considered whether rights may be prioritized and whether claims may carry different moral weight (Ozar, 1985). Some theorists conclude that fundamental moral rights cannot be ranked. Others posit that some fundamental rights must be satisfied before others (Shue, 1980). Thus "basic rights" take precedence over nonbasic rights, which are followed by rights related to cultural enrichment and preference satisfaction. According to this schema, a person must sacrifice any right of lower priority to secure another person's more highly ranked right. Still other theorists suggest ordering rights according to "human needs" (Donnelly, 1985). Each of these approaches offers a theoretical solution, but none addresses the inherent difficulty of defining which rights are basic or which needs are paramount.

A rights-based perspective might view a conflict between rights as a question of whether and how the precedence of one party's right will affect the realization of the right itself. In regard to health, for example, an apparent conflict could be resolved by determining whether and how the protection of either party's right will improve or maintain health.

Consider a hypothetical situation involving the education of children and adolescents about HIV/AIDS prevention measures. Human rights law recognizes the right of parents to determine the education their children receive (UDHR, Art. 26.3) and to assure that their children's religious and moral education conforms with the parents' own (ICESCR, Art. 13.3). Simultaneously, all individuals, including children, possess the right to freedom of opinion and expression and to seek, receive, and impart information and ideas of all kinds (UDHR, Art. 19; ICCPR, Art. 19; Convention on the Rights of the Child, Art. 13).

Most AIDS education programs include campaigns or curricula to prevent new HIV infections among children and adolescents. These programs, funded by the government, school systems, or private organizations, are often presented to schoolchildren. Parents, community groups, or religious leaders may assert that AIDS education and prevention materials that discuss sexuality, drug use, or means to prevent HIV infection, including condoms, conflict with their deeply held religious or moral views. They may wish to ban or censor this material. Thus, the children's right to free exchange of information—including information which could save their lives—directly opposes their parents' rights to educate their children in conformity with certain religious and moral views.

The present human rights system has no easy answer for such situations. Public health personnel might apply some of the ranking principles proposed by rights theorists. In this situation, public health personnel might conclude that censorship of educational messages threatens the children's right to life and choose to offer candid information. They might also conclude that the children's rights to life, health, and the free exchange of information are more "basic" and thus take priority over parents' rights to direct their offsprings' religious and moral instruction. Although grounded in theoretical principles, such a ranking might not persuade the parents and the community, nor improve the working relationship between public health personnel and the community.

Another approach suggests that public health advocates gain the trust and cooperation of the community, parents, and religious leaders in planning and implementing any AIDS prevention effort. The ranking of rights could be used as a starting point in a dialogue between public health and the community. In the best of situations, participation might educate the parents about the threats posed by HIV infection in the community and allow parents' concerns to be addressed in the curriculum's design. Ultimately, however, there may be no way to compromise on some issues, such as condoms. Public health advocates and educators must consider both the relative burdens their policies place on children's and parents' rights and the unintended effects on the community (see Chapters 3 and 4).

Human Rights: Culturally Relative, or Universal and Indivisible?

One of the persistent tensions within human rights doctrine pits respect for cultural differences against a defined set of recognized and protected individual rights. The proposed universality of human rights was hotly debated during the World Conference on Human Rights in 1993; the result was a resounding reaffirmation (Vienna Declaration and Programme of Action, 1993).

Universality, in the context of international human rights, means that all governments must respect a defined set of minimum standards by which to treat individuals within their jurisdictions. Properly defined and understood, universality does not seek to impose a Western conception of civilization, nor does it aim to harmonize or homogenize cultures. The core protections must be observed, but the forms for observance—as long as they adhere to minimum standards—may be adjusted to respect the legal, moral, and cultural systems concerned. Widespread acceptance exists across cultures regarding the validity of certain core rights, as evidenced by broad acceptance of the nonderogable rights identified in the ICCPR (including the right to life, or to be free from slavery, torture, and inhuman treatment). Substantial disagreement exists as to the definition and understanding of other rights.

Widespread ratification of the International Covenants throughout the world suggests a certain level of acceptance of the universal system. Legally, states that have freely assumed treaty-based human rights obligations may not avoid those duties by invoking claims of cultural relativism. Too often, governments rely on cultural relativity to avoid compliance with international obligations. Tolerance of discrimination, enslavement, or genocide, couched in claims of "cultural practice," belie a fundamental misunderstanding of the meaning of cultural relativity. Some governments attack universality in fervent and sometimes violent attempts to suppress domestic movements for democracy, free expression, or self-determination. Such actions are less a demonstration of cultural interpretation of human rights than a desire to maintain control under any circumstances. "Many of the claims made have no foundation whatsoever in such traditions. Instead they reflect no more than the age-old tendency of governments to justify the cynical and self-interested proposition that their own citizens neither want nor need the protection of human rights" (Alston, 1993).

Public health practitioners who seek to incorporate human rights principles into health policy face a challenge: How can they design and implement policies which meet universal human rights norms and still respect the rich variety of traditions and practices of world cultures? For example, where a society that emphasizes group over individual rights seeks to restrict the latter in a manner impermissible under international human rights law, a conflict arises. Traditional practices are not always congruent with international human rights norms in a way that equally respects both.

These conflicts may be particularly problematic in the field of health and human rights because they frequently implicate the long-marginalized rights of discrete subpopulations such as women or religious and ethnic minorities. Evidence suggests that promoting the full realization of the human rights of marginalized groups may be necessary for them to achieve good health. Where "respect" for cultural differences results in conditions which harm the health of disenfranchised groups, special promotion and protection of their rights may be appropriate, even in opposition to cultural or traditional norms. For example, many societies condemn or stigmatize homosexuality. Such stigmatization discourages persons who engage in homosexual activity from seeking or cooperating with preventive health measures or from being honest with health care providers about their sexual behavior. For this reason, public health officials could legitimately oppose such discrimination—even where it has a cultural or religious basis—because it harms public health.

Female genital mutilation, for instance, inflicts well-documented physical and psychological damage to many women and girls (American Medical Association, 1995). The practice increases the risk of complications during childbirth for both mother and child, and, where prevalent, contributes to high maternal and infant mortality and morbidity (Toubia, 1994). The World Health Assembly has called for the elimination of this and other traditional practices which impair women's and children's health (World Health Assembly, 1993). Many women's organizations within Africa are educating about and lobbying against the practice (Dorkenoo, Elworthy, 1992; Helie-Lucas, 1993). The Ghanaian Association on Women's Welfare successfully campaigned to amend the criminal law to include female genital mutilation as a punishable offense. In Kenya, women's rights groups continue efforts to enact and enforce laws to prevent the practice (Kiragu, 1995). Other women, however, criticize Western responses as paternalistic, judgmental, and too narrowly focused on one aspect of discrimination against women (Dawit, Mekuria, 1993; Savand, 1979).

Regardless of the international debate, if local people perceive public health action as culturally insensitive or paternalistic, trust or cooperation between residents and public health personnel will suffer. The result may be counterproductive, alienating the community and the group which the program is designed to help. Public health efforts to change practices that have well-documented negative health consequences need not be designed or perceived as culturally insensitive. For example, campaigns to reduce the incidence of female genital mutilation should strive to achieve the public health goal while minimizing human rights burdens. Effective efforts to achieve this balance might include individual and community education, provision of services in a culturally and linguistically sensitive manner, and continued work to involve local community and religious leaders (Kiragu, 1995) (see chapters 3 and 4).

Where conservative religious traditions restrict women's participation in society at every level—denying girls access to education, barring women from public employment or government participation, discriminating against women in marriage, divorce, and child custody issues—a human rights perspective offers no simple solutions (Cook, 1993).

Questions concerning cultural differences in the definition, scope, or implementation of rights are complex. Unless policymakers adopt an absolutist approach, either insisting on absolute universalism or complete relativism, solutions will require great sensitivity to all aspects of the underlying issue. Factors to consider include, but are not limited to, the following:

1. How fundamental is the right concerned?
2. How important (to the members of the community) is the cultural practice which differs from human rights norms?
3. Is the practice part of an intact cultural system which protects or achieves some of the goals of human rights?
4. Do legitimate cultural leaders support the practice?
5. Do the individuals affected support the practice?
6. Does it negatively impact individuals who are incapable of supporting or opposing it (e.g., children)?

Most importantly perhaps, these questions must be resolved subsequent to a full hearing of the affected parties, following the spread of education and information about the health risks and benefits, and after an attempt has been made to reconcile human rights with respect for genuine cultural differences.

2

Harmonizing Human Rights and Public Health

FROM HUMAN RIGHTS TO PUBLIC HEALTH

International human rights law (human rights, for short) seeks to promote and protect individuals' rights against the state's interference or neglect. The area we refer to as public health, in contrast, encompasses efforts by the state to ensure the conditions under which people can be healthy (Institute of Medicine, 1988) and often includes governmental intervention into individuals' lives to protect the community's health. Thus, the two compete: Human rights protect the rights of individuals, and public health protects the collective good. Evolving approaches to public health, however, emphasize respect for individual rights, trust between public health personnel and the community, conditions of nondiscrimination, and adequate access to health care and education. Often, governmental efforts to promote human rights—including providing social security and adequate health services and restraining from interference with individual liberty and privacy—produce conditions that foster the community's health (IFRC, FXB, 1995).

Some tensions between human rights and public health can be resolved through careful analysis. For example, early in the AIDS pandemic, some governments isolated suspected HIV "carriers," ostensibly compromising personal liberty for the public good. Although the deprivations of freedom violated human rights, they were ineffective in controlling disease transmission. Virtually all public health organizations have concluded that no rational public health justification exists for isolating persons based solely on their HIV status (United Nations, 1996a). Despite a dearth of evidence, however, some countries continue to consider and implement such policies.

Other tensions between human rights and public health seem tenacious, if not intractable. For example, legitimate public health measures, such as surveillance and collection of personal health information, provide accurate, complete, and timely public health and clinical data. Efforts such as named HIV reporting, however, can invade individual privacy. Moreover, unwanted disclosure of results can lead to stigmatization and discrimination. As part of the social contract, individuals may be obliged to forgo a degree of privacy for the community's good (Gostin, 1995b). In turn, society should adopt and enforce measures to safeguard sensitive health information from unjustified dissemination.

Efforts to resolve conflicts between human rights and public health should seek to maximize public health efficacy while minimizing human rights incursions. The human rights impact assessment, introduced in Chapter 3, offers a method by which to balance public health benefits with human rights burdens.

The Relationship Between Health and Human Rights

Recent scholarly writing has probed the relationship between health and human rights (Mann, Gostin, et al., 1994). Several interconnections are listed below.[1]

Public health policies and programs may burden human rights

HIV/AIDS policies implicate a broad range of civil and political, as well as economic, social, and cultural, rights. Both types of rights are essential to human dignity, and both are equally entitled to be considered when formulating HIV/AIDS policies. Most often, governments design and implement public health policies and programs either through legislation that compels or prohibits action by public or private sector actors, or through executive functions (e.g., operating government ministries or offering public services).

Public health measures harbor the potential to negatively or positively impact human rights. States that have ratified one or both of the International Covenants possess a duty to devise policies that promote human rights (Schachter, 1991). Even countries that have not ratified a Covenant, however, may find that protection of human rights may also produce more effective HIV/AIDS policies.

Many public health policies, programs, and activities deeply intrude into people's daily lives (United Nations, 1991, 1992; Tomasevski, Gruskin, et al., 1992). Coercive policies most clearly illustrate this idea. For instance, compulsory medical examinations, immunizations, and testing or treatment violate individuals' security of person unless based on full consent and voluntary cooperation (see Chapter 1: Right to Security). Isolation and quarantine limit liberty and freedom, and, depending upon the conditions of confinement, may constitute inhuman or degrading treatment (see Chapter 1: Freedom of Movement, Freedom from Inhuman and Degrading Treatment).

Even voluntary programs and policies may unjustifiably impinge upon human rights. For example, consider a state program that voluntarily screens for specific health conditions or offers free or low-cost health services, and yet excludes—either explicitly or practically—persons of a certain gender, race, ethnicity, or religious background. Almost all public health programs make distinctions of some kind, but programs that bar persons based upon unreasonable or subjective criteria violate the basic human rights

1. For these, we gratefully acknowledge the contributions of Professor Jonathan Mann and our colleagues at the Harvard School of Public Health.

principle of nondiscrimination (see Chapter 1: Nondiscrimination). Biomedical researchers raise human rights concerns when they neglect to obtain subjects' informed consent, expose them to unreasonable risks, or deny them benefits of medical and technical
innovations (World Health Organization, 1989j; Council of International Organizations
of Medical Sciences (CIOMS), 1991, 1993; see also Chapter 4: Research on Human
Subjects).

Rigorous evaluation of public health policies, then, demands at least two types of
assessment. The first is traditionally undertaken in public health scholarship and practice: determining whether a program cost-effectively improves health outcomes. The
second is often neglected by public health practitioners: assessing the program's human
rights impact on individuals and groups. These two areas of analysis—public health and
human rights—are not mutually exclusive, but often exist in alliance; programs which
respect human rights often advance health outcomes, and programs that impede human
rights tend to hinder public health objectives (IFRC, FXB, 1995; see Chapter 3).

Human rights abuses often measurably harm health

Frequently, human rights violations negatively affect health. Egregious violations (e.g.,
torture) can inflict pain, disfigurement, and even death. During recent decades, a growing number of countries have ratified the major human rights instruments, yet many
continue to practice or permit gross human rights violations (Human Rights Watch, 1995;
Amnesty International, 1993, 1984).

Physicians, forensic pathologists, psychiatrists, and others have examined human
rights violations and their effects (Geiger, Cook-Deegan, 1993; Swiss, Giller, 1993;
Sandler, Epstein, et al., 1991; Harvard Study Team, 1991). Research methods include
examining detainees or prisoners for signs of torture or mistreatment; exhuming individual or mass graves; conducting autopsies to determine and document the cause of
death and details of mistreatment; employing epidemiological methods to calculate the
effects of infrastructure destruction on child morbidity and mortality; assessing the psychological sequela of violent events on survivors; and testing for environmental evidence of biological or chemical warfare. Research has also found long-term psychological consequences of human rights violations. For instance, torture, rape, and other
traumatic events (e.g., imprisonment, deprivation of food or water, bombing or shell-
ing, or witnessing a neighbor or family member's assault or murder) are associated with
prolonged and severe psychological trauma in both children and adults (Basoglu, Paker,
et al., 1994; Mollica, Donelan, et al., 1993; Mollica, Caspi-Yavin, 1991).

Human rights violations can occur during times of war or peace, although those committed during the latter may not fit the model of gross human rights abuses and may be
more difficult to discern. In some societies, for example, a woman cannot seek or consent to medical treatment without her husband's or father's approval. A pregnant woman
in labor whose husband or father is absent may die or suffer severe complications while
awaiting his return (Prevention of Maternal Mortality Network, 1990). Here, gender
discrimination undergirds the resulting illness, death, and disability (see Chapter 1:

Nondiscrimination). But these violations are not limited to the developing world. Research revealed that in Baltimore, Maryland, African Americans diagnosed with HIV were less likely than whites to receive antiretroviral medication, leaving them at greater risk for opportunistic infection and physical deterioration (Moore, Stanton, et al., 1994). If further investigation suggests that racial bias is at the root of disparate medical treatment, one might suspect unjustified discrimination.

State censorship of HIV educational materials, or restrictions of messages in specific media, may deprive individuals of the information necessary to protect them from HIV. Where such censorship unjustifiably interferes with the free exchange of information, it violates the freedom to seek, receive, and impart information. Such infringement may increase vulnerability to disease, infection, morbidity, and mortality.

Promoting human rights is critical to improving health

At times, health promotion depends upon human rights protection. For example, interventions that trample the rights of discrete groups tend to be disempowering; persons may lose the means, if not the will, to protect themselves from health threats. In contrast, recognizing rights can enable people to benefit their own health.

Consider the effects of AIDS prevention strategies among women. Due to underlying social conditions, many women are unable or unwilling to engage in safer sex. Where women are economically and socially dependent on men—or are required or expected to defer to their wishes—women are less able to protect themselves from HIV (Hamblin, Reid, 1991). Promoting women's full and equal access to and enjoyment of basic human rights (e.g., education, adequate standard of living, equal employment opportunity, equal rights during and after marriage, access to necessary medical care, and safety and security of person) is not only worthwhile but promotes women's ability to protect themselves from disease.

Similarly, certain groups that are disproportionately burdened by disease tend to be also routinely denied basic human rights. For example, poverty is associated with increased mortality and morbidity (Pappas, Queen, et al., 1993). Yet, greater access to health services may not be the only way to reduce the negative health impact of low income. Research is needed to investigate the relationship between poverty and poor health. To lower morbidity and mortality may require promoting men's, women's, and children's rights (e.g., nondiscrimination and the rights to education and to work in a safe and healthful setting)—offering an escape from poverty and a path to greater productivity and employability.

How the human rights and public health framework are complementary

Government efforts to protect the public health often limit individuals' rights and liberties. Beginning with the Universal Declaration, human rights instruments have allowed limits on individual exercise and enjoyment of some rights if necessary to protect the "general welfare" (UDHR, Art. 29.2; ICESCR, Art. 4; ICCPR, Art. 18, 19, 21, 22).

The broad discretion granted to government officials by these instruments is not, however, limitless. As the ICCPR and the Siracusa Principles set forth, any restrictions of the Covenant's rights must be strictly provided by law, neither arbitrary nor discriminatory, based on objective considerations, necessary to respond to a pressing social need enumerated in the text (which includes public health), proportional to the social aim, and no more restrictive than necessary to achieve the intended purpose (Siracusa Principles, 1984). These criteria can guide public health officials in determining the circumstances in which to limit human rights articulated in both the ICCPR and the ICESCR.

Public health officials, and those who define or implement public health policies, bear a heavy burden. To protect the public health, they possess the power and authority to intrude into private activities of people's daily lives and can infringe upon the full range of individual rights and freedoms. To exercise their power appropriately, public health and other government officials must act in conformity with domestic and international norms and human rights systems. Chapter 3 suggests a step-by-step analysis for applying human rights norms to public health policies, programs, or activities.

By carefully examining public health policies through the lens of human rights, policymakers can often eliminate or modify unduly burdensome measures. For example, one can examine compulsory detention, isolation, or quarantine based on public health grounds under the domestic legal standards of due process and equal protection. In countries that constitutionally or statutorily proscribe racial discrimination, public health proposals which target or exclude racial minorities from programs or services are susceptible to legal challenges permitted under domestic law. Domestic remedies and enforcement systems remain the primary and most expeditious means to enforce human rights violations (Bilder, 1986). Unfortunately, many countries' domestic remedies are inadequate, unenforceable, or nonexistent.

International human rights norms provide a uniform standard of rights and responsibilities designed to foster respect for the individual. International and regional human rights systems offer a forum in which to evaluate and adjudicate claims of human rights violations at a distance from domestic circumstances (Shelton, 1986; Drzemczewski, 1983; see also Chapter 1). Reporting, monitoring, and adjudication within the international system, with all of its inherent weaknesses, increases the visibility of human rights and exerts public pressure on nations that do not want to be publicly recognized for having committed human rights abuses (Bilder, 1986). The conclusion by an international body that a country is violating human rights can encourage other states to respond with condemnation, sanctions, or even direct action.

Furthermore, acceptance of "rights language" and a human rights approach may help to shift the health dialogue. Such a shift is imperative in crafting HIV/AIDS policy to encourage governments to eschew coercive policies that control disease by controlling those infected, and to harness state power and resources to create the conditions in which people can be healthy (Institute of Medicine, 1988).

Government health initiatives are often constrained by financial resources and viewed as secondary to political, ideological, or cultural concerns. However, "when a society recognizes that a person has a right, it affirms, legitimates, and justifies that entitlement, and incorporates and establishes it in the society's system of values giving it important weight in competition with other societal values" (Henkin, 1990). Raising the profile of health issues on governmental agendas by linking them to human rights could enable individuals or groups to initiate more effective government health policies.

Health advocates have proposed a rights-based approach to health in contexts other than the HIV/AIDS pandemic. Increasingly, human rights are connected to the rights and status of women in society; the interrelationships between women's rights and population policies are particularly strong (World Health Organization, 1993c; Tomasevski, 1994; Sen, Germain, et al., 1994; Sen, Snow, 1994).

In a paper presented to the ECOSOC, the American Association for the Advancement of Science (AAAS) posited a number of positive effects that a human rights approach can have on the right to health (United Nations, 1993a):

> 1) emphasizes the equality of all persons and their inherent right to health as the foundation of the health-care system;
>
> 2) conveys the idea that health, and state action to promote and protect health, are fundamentally important social goods and should be considered differently from other goods and services;
>
> 3) focuses particularly on the needs of the most disadvantaged and vulnerable communities (embracing both nondiscrimination and affirmative efforts to correct historical inequities);
>
> 4) balances individual needs with the common good, making the viability and effectiveness of the public health (and health) sector a shared concern and responsibility;
>
> 5) creates state obligations both to protect individual rights relevant to health (security of person, right to free exchange of information) and to provide certain levels of services or support necessary for good health (such as universal primary education, social security, childhood immunizations, maternal and child health services);
>
> 6) empowers individuals to assert their claims by creating clear individual entitlements to state protection or provision of benefits;
>
> 7) underscores the importance of public participation in setting priorities, monitoring public policies, and operating health sector institutions; and
>
> 8) provides potential recourse for those who experience violations.

Each of these goals might be achieved through another perspective on health (e.g., ethics, domestic law, psychology, or economics). As presented here, human rights offers an approach based on human dignity, fundamental liberty, and entitlement that transcends national and disciplinary borders and suggests that systemic health problems call for a deeper understanding of societal inequities.

Thus, health and human rights are tightly intertwined. Public health programs can negatively or positively affect human rights, and human rights abuses in times of conflict or peace can measurably impact health. Applying a human rights framework to health can help refocus public debate from reliance on coercive policies toward fully realizing human health and well-being.

A FOCUS ON AIDS IN HUMAN RIGHTS

The International Bill of Rights and regional human rights accords do not mention AIDS, and international human rights enforcement agencies have rarely dealt with violations of HIV-infected individuals' rights. Nonetheless, an array of international resolutions and recommendations explicitly address AIDS and human rights. Although not legally binding, these documents represent the international public health and human rights communities' broad consensus regarding the rights of persons living with HIV/AIDS and the interdependency of human rights and public health. These instruments illustrate the many ways in which human rights and public health are integral to fighting the AIDS pandemic.

In May 1987, the United Nations Fortieth World Health Assembly first officially recognized the need for international cooperation in research and education about AIDS. Since then, the World Health Assembly, WHO's Global Programme on AIDS (now UNAIDS), and many international public health organizations, human rights groups, and NGOs have passed resolutions concerning the prevention and control of the HIV pandemic. Many public health policies and consensus statements from the World Health Organization, for example, highlight the importance of human rights principles. The subject of these documents ranges from transmission of HIV infection (World Health Organization, 1987b) by sexual behavior (World Health Organization, 1989c–e) or needle sharing (World Health Organization, 1988c) to screening (World Health Organization, 1987c,d, 1992h), the role of sexually transmitted infections (World Health Organization, 1992f), pregnancy and breast-feeding (World Health Organization/UNICEF, 1992), international travel and migration (World Health Organization, 1987d, 1988e), prisons (World Health Organization, 1987e, 1993b), and the workplace (World Health Organization, 1988f, 1991b).

Space precludes presenting the entire array of AIDS-specific documents relevant to human rights. Instead, we present four broad themes that emerge from AIDS-specific resolutions: (1) The *global AIDS strategy* should reflect a deep respect for human rights; (2) national policies should follow a *voluntary approach* which values autonomy, cooperation, and consent; (3) persons with HIV infection or AIDS possess the right to *privacy* and confidentiality of health care information; and (4) persons with HIV infection or AIDS have the right to be free from invidious *discrimination*.

The Global AIDS Strategy

On several occasions, the World Health Assembly has endorsed the World Health Organization's global strategy to prevent and control AIDS. In 1987, 1989, and 1992, the Assembly urged the development of global strategies and programs to combat AIDS and encouraged cooperation at all levels—national, regional, and international—through the sharing of programs, technology, and information (World Health Organization, 1992c,d).

The United Nations General Assembly (1988, 1989a) strengthened global cooperation in the AIDS pandemic by supporting NGOs' efforts and national policies to assist women, children, and intravenous drug users. The General Assembly stressed that programs are needed to improve the public's understanding of and attitude toward persons with HIV infection or AIDS. Regional, national, and global AIDS strategies should reflect a deep respect for human rights (World Health Organization, 1988a).

UNAIDS, the interagency program which coordinates HIV/AIDS efforts within the United Nations system, has adopted protection and promotion of human rights as one of its core principles and as a foundation for its strategic plan of action (United Nations [UNAIDS], 1995e, 1996).

Voluntarism in AIDS Prevention and Control Strategies

Autonomy, cooperation, and consent

Harmonizing human rights and public health requires a voluntaristic approach wherever possible. Policies that value autonomy, cooperation, and consent protect individuals' rights while improving communities' welfare. The World Health Organization report on social aspects of AIDS (1987a), the International Consultation on Health Legislation and Ethics in Oslo (1988), and the United Nations Centre for Human Rights Consultation on AIDS and Human Rights in Geneva (1989b) recognize this theme. In addition, the Council of Europe (1987, 1989a,b) and the European Parliament (1989) have specifically endorsed this approach.

Some argue that coercive measures (e.g., compulsory testing, isolation, or criminal prosecutions) are necessary to fight a lethal disease that is spread by elective behaviors. Indeed, coercive measures may prevent a few cases of transmission, but for several reasons, they are unlikely to reduce the overall prevalence of HIV infection in the population. First, individuals' fear of and resistance to compulsory measures impede attempts to educate and counsel people on safer sexual and needle-sharing behaviors. Coercion may drive persons with HIV or AIDS away from needed services. Thus, compulsory measures may increase seroprevalence—just the opposite result intended.

Second, governments often apply coercive powers in a discriminatory fashion by targeting poor people, racial or ethnic minorities, or other disfavored populations. For example, a decision by a government to "get tough" on commercial sex workers often ignores the men who market and use the women's services (World Health Organization, 1989c).

Third, compulsory measures often inefficiently divert valuable resources from AIDS services. For example, mandatory screening of a large population can be costly and may fail to reduce HIV infection rates. Similarly, depriving a person of liberty in a health care facility or prison requires inordinate expenditures for housing, food, clothing, and treatment. Instead, directing resources to counseling and education and a broad range of services (e.g., housing, social services, nutrition, and medical treatment, including treatment for drug dependency) may be far more effective. Based on these disadvantages, international opinion rejects the simplistic idea that coercive measures promote public health.

A voluntaristic approach encompasses the elements of autonomy, consent, and cooperation. To empower individuals and help communities effect voluntary changes, AIDS policies should be formulated in cooperation with the affected populations and implemented with respect for individual autonomy. Developing strategies in close consultation with the communities affected enables policymakers to ensure the local population's participation in prevention and treatment programs. By respecting autonomy and requiring informed consent, public officials encourage people to come forward as valued members of the society.

Clearly, voluntarism in AIDS policy is neither simple nor universally accepted. Hard questions have been asked: Why exempt HIV/AIDS from the coercive measures traditionally adopted for other infectious diseases such as tuberculosis or sexually transmitted diseases (Bayer, 1991; Burris, 1994)? Nor is it necessarily wrong for governments to penalize or restrict obviously dangerous behavior recklessly or willfully undertaken. Nevertheless, a broad base of public health opinion holds that voluntaristic approaches such as education, testing with consent, and counseling are most likely to be effective. Proponents of this approach argue that HIV should be dealt with differently because it is transmitted differently than, say, tuberculosis (e.g., airborne transmission). Moreover, a discernable transformation of opinion has occurred among public health authorities concerning the efficacy of compulsion. Many public health theorists now believe that past uses of compulsion have not worked as well as previously thought in impeding the spread of disease epidemics (Brandt, 1987).

Confidentiality and Privacy

Numerous statements by the WHO (1989b), the Council of Europe (1987, 1989b), the United Nations Commission on Human Rights (1995a, 1994a), and UNAIDS (United Nations, 1996a) endorse the core principles of privacy and confidentiality. For example, WHO recommends that casefinding programs respect confidentiality in collecting information about individuals and populations through testing or screening (World Health Organization, 1987c, 1988d), partner notification (World Health Organization, 1989d), and epidemiological research (World Health Organization, 1989a; CIOMS, 1991).

Not only is safeguarding individual privacy a primary ethical responsibility of health care professionals, it is also necessary to effectively provide health services. A sphere of privacy surrounds each person's relationship with health care professionals. Persons living with HIV/AIDS have a particularly strong interest in preserving the confidentiality of health care information that concerns the most private parts of their lives (e.g., sexual relationships or injecting drug use). If revealed, this information may harm the person's work, family, and community status.

Maintaining confidentiality serves the public health because it encourages people to speak candidly with doctors, nurses, counselors, healers, and public health officials. Ensuring confidentiality and encouraging cooperation can foster changes in behavior and healthier choices by individuals and communities.

Privacy and public health, of course, are not always in consonance. In societies that collect and use information for the public good, some tradeoffs between privacy and public health may be inevitable. Many public health activities regarded as effective (e.g., epidemiological surveillance, research, and reporting) potentially invade privacy. In its own way, each public health practice may involve the collection, storage, and use of identifiable information by government or the private sector. Provided these data are essential to achieving public health purposes, are maintained in secure systems, and are not reused in ways that stigmatize or discriminate, the common good may outweigh the minimal privacy invasions.

Nondiscrimination

In AIDS-specific resolutions, the right to be free from discrimination has received the greatest attention (see, e.g., World Health Organization, 1989b; Council of Europe, 1989a,b; United Nations, 1996a, 1995a,b, 1994a,b). The Forty-first World Health Assembly (1988) urged member states to protect from discrimination persons with HIV infection or AIDS. Moreover, the Assembly recommended that national programs foster a spirit of understanding and compassion by providing information, education, and social support programs, and it encouraged states to protect the rights and inherent dignity of individuals; to avoid stigmatization and discrimination in services, employment, and travel; and to ensure confidentiality in counseling and testing.

The World Health Assembly endorsed the historic London Declaration on AIDS Prevention adopted by the World Summit of Ministers in 1988. The London Declaration emphasized "the need in AIDS prevention programmes to protect human rights and human dignity. Discrimination against, and stigmatization of, HIV-infected people and people with AIDS and population groups undermine public health and must be avoided."

Four reports highlight the preeminence of the nondiscrimination principle in international human rights law. In July 1989, the International Consultation on AIDS and Human Rights met in Geneva (United Nations Centre for Human Rights, 1989b). The group observed that the adverse social, cultural, and political reaction to AIDS threatened to overshadow its public health impact. Reiterating the public health rationale for policies of nondiscrimination, the Consultation noted that HIV is transmitted primarily through behavior that is private, often hidden, and, in some societies, unlawful. Persons who fear severe personal consequences of discriminatory policies will avoid contact with public health programs. "The net result would be to jeopardize seriously educational outreach and thereby exacerbate the difficulty of preventing HIV infection."

In May 1991, in the Hague, the International Movement for the Promotion and Realization of Human Rights and Responsibilities developed the Humanity Declaration and Charter on HIV and AIDS (Rights and Humanity Declaration, 1992). The Declaration and Charter asserts that human rights and principles of ethics and humanity are essential to confront the AIDS pandemic. The Declaration and Charter calls for governments to respect the rights to life, to the highest attainable standard of health, to dignity irrespective of health status, to freedom without unjustified restriction, and to economic assistance for developing countries.

The United Nations Commission on Human Rights invited the Sub-Commission on Prevention of Discrimination and Protection of Minorities to examine the problem of discrimination against persons living with HIV/AIDS (United Nations, 1989c–e). The interim and final reports to the Sub-Commission by Special Rapporteur Luis Varela Quiros coherently analyze the diverse forms of discrimination. Mr. Quiros also surveyed the various means by which governments discriminate against persons living with HIV/AIDS (United Nations, 1991, 1992, 1993), ranging from coercive measures (e.g., restrictions on movement and travel) to victimization of gays, women, and injecting drug users.

In 1994, the Commission on Human Rights requested that the Secretary-General prepare a report on international and domestic measures to protect human rights and prevent discrimination in the HIV/AIDS context, and to submit recommendations. The Secretary-General's report, presented in December of 1994 (United Nations, 1995c), recounted the Commission's actions directing member states to ensure that their laws, policies, and practices—including those related to HIV/AIDS—respect human rights, and asked member states to submit information about international and domestic measures adopted and implemented to protect human rights. The report also reviewed the impact of HIV/AIDS-related discrimination. It noted that discrimination infringes on fundamental individual rights, contributes to the vulnerability of various populations, including women and children, and hampers effective public health efforts to combat the spread of AIDS.

On the international level, the report concluded that HIV/AIDS-related discrimination violates numerous international declarations, covenants, and treaties, and long-standing policies of United Nations–affiliated organizations (e.g., the International Labor Organization [ILO], the United Nations Development Programme [UNDP], the United Nations High Commissioner for Refugees [UNHCR], and the World Health Organization). The Commission on Human Rights and its Sub-Commission confirmed that HIV/AIDS-related discrimination violates existing international law (United Nations, 1995a,b).

On the domestic level, the report described national legislation, policies, and actions that were reported to the Secretary-General. These included national policies (Zimbabwe, The Netherlands), institutional structures (Canada, Mexico, Croatia), education and information programs (New Zealand, Australia, Brazil), and other actions by international NGOs and governments. The report concluded that while many countries in principle reject HIV/AIDS-related discrimination, a "dramatic gap [exists] . . . between national policies and legislation and their implementation." Despite international and national provisions condemning discrimination, coercive policies persist (e.g., involuntary testing; public disclosure of status; segregation; and denial of employment, housing, education, and travel). The report urged member states "to include in the national AIDS programmes specific measures to combat social stigmatization, discrimination and violence directed against persons with HIV/AIDS and to develop a supportive legal and social environment necessary for the effective prevention and care of [persons with] AIDS." To achieve this, all governments should review their legal systems, laws, policies, and practices to ensure that effective antidiscrimination provisions can and are implemented (United Nations, 1995c).

The international community has strongly denounced discrimination against women and children with HIV infection. The United Nations Secretary-General has observed that women's status in many societies "causes them to be more vulnerable to the consequences of AIDS-related discrimination" (United Nations, 1989f, 1995c; see also resolutions of the Human Rights Commission, United Nations, 1994a, 1995a). Women face a heightened risk of HIV infection and discrimination because they disproportionately suffer from poverty, prostitution, and subordination. The Paris Declaration on Women, Children and AIDS (1989), recognizing the depth and pervasiveness of discrimination against women and children, called for enhancing their social, economic, and legal status and respecting their human rights and dignity.

Discrimination against persons living with HIV/AIDS is rooted in the fear of a fatal disease that cannot be adequately treated; the belief that sexual behavior is private, hidden, and, in some societies, unlawful; and the history of deprecation of homosexuals, sex workers, and injecting drug users (IDUs) in many cultures (Merson, 1992). The rights of persons living with HIV/AIDS deserve high priority because they are closely linked to global health. If HIV infection continues to produce stigma and discrimination (e.g., loss of employment, education, or housing, and forced separation from family), then "persons will actively avoid detection, and contact with health and social services will be lost" (World Health Organization, 1988b).

CONCLUSION: THE ROLE OF LAW IN THE HIV PANDEMIC

Ideally, domestic law would promote effective policies that impede HIV transmission while assuring the dignity of each individual living with HIV/AIDS. Unfortunately, many national laws violate the principles enunciated in AIDS-specific human rights documents. To conform with international law, national legislation should be based on sound scientific data—not presupposition, prejudice, and stereotype—and should respect human rights and empower individuals to protect themselves against HIV infection.

The president, prime minister, and chief justice of India, in endorsing the New Delhi Declaration and Action Plan on HIV/AIDS (6–10 December, 1995), set forth the following legal objectives: (1) promote voluntary behavior to protect the health of individuals, families, and children; (2) prevent coercive and punitive action against persons living with HIV/AIDS; (3) protect society and promote a sense of individual responsibility; (4) facilitate access to information, health care, and legal services to promote health and protect rights; and (5) allocate adequate resources for prevention, care, and antidiscrimination—including support for government and nongovernmental organizations and networks of people living with HIV/AIDS.

Despite striking differences in culture, in economic resources, and in social perspectives between North and South, and East and West, and despite differences in the history, language, and approach of the human rights and public health communities, many now perceive a potent public health/human rights synergy in the arena of the AIDS pandemic. Alone, respect for human rights will not ensure public health. To achieve aspirations for public health and human rights, society must carefully examine its duties to promote public health, to respect human dignity, and to empower vulnerable persons to protect themselves. The question then arises: Which health policies most effectively promote health while least restricting human rights? The next chapter offers an organizational tool to answer that question—the human rights impact assessment.

3

Human Rights Impact Assessment[1]

Policymakers often rely upon public health necessity or benefit to justify policies or programs that limit human rights. Protection of the public health is a legitimate reason for restricting certain rights. The power to narrow rights, however, must be exercised judiciously and is subject to the requirements established in the primary human rights documents (UDHR, Art. 29; ICCPR, Art. 4; ICESCR, Art. 4) and statements that prescribe specific standards by which states may limit individual rights (Siracusa Principles, 1984; United Nations, 1989b, 1990).

Generally, restrictions on human rights must be (1) *prescribed by law in a democratic society*—based upon the genuinely elected legislature's thoughtful consideration, and (2) *necessary to protect a valued social goal*—promoting a compelling public interest (e.g., safety or health).

Limitations on human rights should not be taken lightly. At the same time, government is obligated to protect the public health and promote the general welfare. This chapter presents a "human rights impact assessment," which is a method of analyzing public health policies and programs to ensure that they constitute beneficial public health strategies that do not unduly burden human rights.

Public health officials sometimes craft HIV strategies without carefully considering (1) the goals, (2) whether the means adopted can achieve them, and (3) whether the financial and human rights burdens outweigh the intended benefits. Public health policies have not clearly and systematically integrated international human rights norms. Moreover, few public health officials are familiar with human rights doctrines, and those who are may lack the means to assess a policy from a human rights perspective. Imple-

---

1. The Human Rights Impact Assessment, first published in 1994 (Gostin, Mann), grew out of our work with a group of colleagues at the Harvard School of Public Health, chiefly Dr. Jonathan Mann, Dr. Katarina Tomasevski, and Ms. Sofia Gruskin. The Human Rights Impact Assessment evolved from our collective experience teaching public health, law, and medical students about the relationship between public health and human rights. The goal of the Human Rights Impact Assessment is to provide public health practitioners and others interested in health policy with a systematic approach to exploring the human rights dimensions of public health policies, practices, programs, and resource allocation decisions. The Impact Assessment has been used by students in our classes on human rights and public health at the Harvard School of Public Health and the Georgetown/Johns Hopkins University Program in Law and Public Health.

menting AIDS policies without seriously considering the human rights dimension may
harm those persons affected and undermine the public health strategies themselves
Indeed, no magic formula exists for simultaneously producing a perfect public healt￼
strategy and a model human rights policy. But the basic steps set forth here should hel￼
policymakers to balance competing interests and to develop public health policies tha￼
are both effective and respectful of human rights.

SEVEN-STEP PROCESS FOR ANALYZING PUBLIC HEALTH POLICIES AND PROGRAMS

Find the Facts

Scientists understand the importance of painstakingly gathering and assessing all rel￼
evant facts before drawing a conclusion. The unbiased collection of data by the science
of public health (e.g., epidemiology, virology, bacteriology, immunology, and biosta￼
tistics) and health care (e.g., medicine, nursing, and social services) forms the founda￼
tion for ethical policy development. Assessing a policy's impact on human rights re￼
quires equally rigorous and impartial data collection. Although institutions that seek ￼
justify a policy (such as Ministries of Health or Justice) may present credible argumen￼
ostensibly based upon reliable evidence, their facts nonetheless may be incomplete ￼
biased. Proper fact-finding entails broad-based consultations with other than gover￼
ment actors. For example, international and nonprofit organizations, public health ￼
other professional associations, community-based or advocacy groups, and communi￼
leaders (e.g., elders or tribal leaders) may be invaluable resources in determining ho￼
health policies may affect human rights in their communities. Discussions with HI￼
infected individuals and their advocates are particularly important since the polici￼
directly and intimately impact them. To ensure a balanced picture, public health officia￼
should systematically and comprehensively gather material from diverse viewpoint
    After the fact-finding process, AIDS policy analysis can begin. The human righ￼
impact assessment offers a step-by-step series of questions designed to balance publ￼
health benefits against human rights burdens.

Determine if the Public Health Purpose Is Compelling

Human rights assessment cannot occur in a vacuum. Policymakers must possess a tho￼
ough understanding of the intended public health purposes, which are no less than co￼
pelling. Even a powerful public health justification does not warrant disregard of hum￼
rights. Most policies in some way affect autonomy, privacy, or equality. Serious incu￼
sions of human rights (e.g., liberty or freedom from inhuman and degrading treatme￼
weigh heavily in a balance of interests.

First, public health officials must define the problem; a clear conceptualization will help to craft more carefully tailored policies. A general claim that the goal "is to combat AIDS" is vague and overbroad. More narrowly defined public health goals include (1) initiating specific behavioral changes (e.g., decreasing unprotected homosexual or heterosexual intercourse, or the sharing of contaminated drug injection equipment), (2) improving occupational safety (e.g., enhancing compliance with infection control standards), or (3) safeguarding the blood supply (e.g., through serological screening).

The objective should be consistent with a country's or region's priorities and epidemiology. For example, consider a developing country where epidemiological evidence demonstrates that HIV is transmitted mainly through heterosexual behavior or needle sharing. To expend a large portion of state resources to minimize the occurrence of unprotected intercourse between men would not help achieve the most compelling public health goal. Moreover, such a policy might drain scarce resources and divert public attention from behaviors that are transmitting HIV in the area.

Requiring policymakers to define their goals clearly and critically ensures a valid public health objective and facilitates public debate. Furthermore, this exercise may expose prejudices, stereotypical attitudes, and irrational fears and may safeguard against policies that, for example, unfairly target disenfranchised groups (e.g., commercial sex workers, foreigners, or ethnic minorities).

Evaluate How Effectively the Policy Would Achieve the Public Health Purpose

A valid, or even compelling, public health objective does not in itself justify an AIDS policy. Public officials should carry the burden of showing that the proposed means are reasonably likely to achieve the stated purpose. This requires an honest, rigorous scientific investigation. Policymakers should evaluate the strategy by every tool available— impartially examining the facts and expert opinion, and fully consulting with affected groups—and abandon policies that appear fundamentally flawed. Public officials should evaluate alternative solutions with the same careful scrutiny.

Developing appropriate questions is one of the most important steps in determining the efficacy of an AIDS policy. Not every policy requires the same questions; however, a useful set of questions will enable policymakers to better evaluate other strategies.

The following questions, applied to HIV screening as an example, offer a guide with which to systematically evaluate AIDS policies (Brandt, Cleary, et al., 1990; Gostin, 1986).

Is the form of intervention appropriate and accurate?

To estimate the potential benefits and harms of any intervention, the policymaker must know its accuracy. In screening programs, three distinct sources of error exist: (1) testing during the "window" period (after HIV infection but before HIV antibodies are detectable); (2) testing under adverse conditions, variations in test kits, and human error; and (3) the prevalence of HIV infection in the target population.

Screening programs in large populations with predictably low frequencies of infection (such as premarital screening in most countries) are flawed in several ways. They unnecessarily invade the privacy of many people, consume scarce resources, and identify relatively few infected individuals. In addition, the positive predictive value (PPV) of the test in a population with a low level of infection is relatively low. Generally, the lower the prevalence of HIV infection in a particular population, the smaller the probability that a positive result is accurate, and the greater the probability that it constitutes a "false positive." Even with a test as sensitive and specific as an HIV-antibody test, the predictive accuracy still depends on the proportion of persons tested who are infected (Cleary, Barry, et al., 1987). The technical capability of the tests cannot, therefore, be separated from the specific context in which they are used (World Health Organization, 1992h).

Is the intervention likely to lead to effective action?

Initiation of a screening, partner notification, or isolation program does not necessarily mean that the program is worthwhile. The issue is whether the program is effective.

In regard to screening programs, policymakers must first determine the marginal value of test results: That is, given what is already known about the patient or population, does the test yield new, useful information? More importantly, does the policy utilize that information productively? These questions suggest that one will pursue routine testing only if it leads to preventing HIV transmission or to providing health care not otherwise accessible. Screening and testing, then, emerge as effective public health programs only if the information collected is used to benefit the individual or to promote the public health.

Some policymakers contend that gathering information about HIV status in a population is always, in itself, beneficial. Governments sometimes use epidemiological data derived from testing or screening programs to chart an epidemic's course, allocate present or future resources, or appeal for international assistance. However, experts often challenge the validity or applicability of data that are not obtained through scientifically designed protocols. Thus, the potential harms of such data may overwhelm the benefits, particularly where individual identities are disclosed. Moreover, alone, collection or dissemination of the results of testing or screening will not bring about behavioral change. To effect long-lasting behavior change among communities and individuals at risk requires well-tailored programs for education and counseling.

Has the person consented?

Legal and ethical standards strongly suggest that public health programs incorporate the principle of informed consent. This doctrine applies in many contexts, including contact tracing, treatment, biomedical research, and HIV testing when a person's identity can be ascertained. Informed consent rests upon respect for personal autonomy and privacy. The principle of autonomy recognizes that every competent human being has the right to make decisions regarding her health and well-being. Privacy principles include the right to maintain the confidentiality of intimate information (see Chapter 1: Right to Security; Privacy).

Professional standards of care hold informed consent in high regard. Health care providers consider consent as a dynamic process of communication and interaction with the patient rather than an inert legal concept. The process of consent offers an opportunity to counsel and educate, preserves the integrity of the caregiver–patient relationship, and acknowledges the patient's dignity.

Looking at AIDS policies in a new way: will a particular policy be as effective as other policies (opportunity costs)?

To evaluate whether a policy achieves the intended public health goal, public officials should examine the policy through a lens that is new to the human rights framework— that of "opportunity costs." This step involves comparing a proposed policy to potential alternatives and may help policymakers learn whether an initially desirable program is in fact less effective and more invasive than another approach. For example, one purpose of screening is to effect behavioral change. A confidential program of counseling and education, however, could achieve the same goal without the privacy invasions imposed by population screening.

This comparative approach encourages public health officials to examine all policies with a fresh perspective. For instance, certain populations (e.g., commercial sex workers and people who have multiple sex partners) are often targeted for mandatory screening (Tomasevski, Gruskin, et al., 1992). Coercive or punitive interventions alienate these communities and fuel the very behaviors that the policies seek to prevent. Instead, health officials might investigate how to empower women and men who are unable to refuse sexual intercourse or demand that their partners use a condom. Public officials might also work to meet women and children's employment, housing, health, and social needs to promote their dignity and minimize their exploitation.

Public policy is a tool to improve community health. A hasty decision to initiate a comprehensive program of screening, contact tracing, or coercive measures imposes more than financial and human rights burdens. It exacts opportunity costs. Devoting resources to one policy necessarily deprives a government of the opportunity to introduce other potentially more effective policies or services. The global community can ill afford to forgo cost-effective measures that prevent HIV infection and promote access to care.

In sum, to evaluate policy options, policymakers should ask several questions: Is the form of intervention appropriate and accurate? Is the intervention likely to lead to effective action? Will the policy elicit the consent and cooperation of those affected? Is a particular policy as effective as other feasible options? Public health officials who deliberate over these and other questions are most likely to reduce the overall prevalence of HIV infection in their populations while respecting human rights.

Determine Whether the Public Health Policy Is Well-Targeted

Once public officials conclude that a policy would effectively promote the public health, they should consider how to implement it. Well-conceived policies target the population in need. Ideally, policymakers will narrowly tailor their approaches to only those persons who will benefit from them, rather than unnecessarily expending resources and indiscriminately interfering in peoples' lives.

Every policy creates a class of people to whom the policy applies and a class to whom it does not. For example, screening policies may target health care professionals, patients, marriage applicants, newborns, or foreigners. Similarly, criminal penalties may apply only to injecting drug users or commercial sex workers but not to others who engage in high-risk behavior.

Policies that appear neutral may, in fact, disproportionately burden certain groups. For example, programs that automatically isolate persons with tuberculosis who do not complete the full course of treatment may disproportionately burden poor persons who have inadequate access to health care, housing, or transportation. Awareness of this notion will sensitize policymakers to human rights concerns and help to ensure that they create classifications that are related to the public health. Policies that target individuals because of their race, sex, religion, national origin, sexual orientation, economic status, or homelessness are often based on invidious stereotypes.

In addition, policymakers should guard against under- and overinclusion. A policy that is underinclusive reaches some, but not all, of the persons it should. By itself, underinclusion does not pose a human rights problem. Without violating human rights, a government may justifiably allocate limited resources to address a public health problem incrementally. An example of a gradual approach is a government's provision of special HIV prevention and treatment services to street children but not to injecting drug users (IDUs). The underinclusiveness of this policy does not necessarily reflect discrimination; it may simply reflect a particular country's public health priorities.

On the other hand, some underinclusive policies may mask discrimination. For example, providing services to or conducting clinical trials on men but not women, or for heterosexuals but not homosexuals, may reflect animus rather than legitimate priorities. A government's use of its coercive powers to target politically powerless groups, but not others that engage in similar behavior, may indicate discrimination. In designing public health programs, policymakers should check for underinclusiveness (either intentional or unintentional) that decreases the effectiveness of policies or unfairly burdens human rights.

Overinclusion, or overbreadth, occurs when a policy extends to more people than necessary to achieve the objective. Overbreadth in the provision of benefits does not violate human rights, although it may not be cost-effective. For example, counseling or educating persons who are unlikely to engage in high-risk behaviors is consistent with human rights principles but likely to be costly and perhaps unnecessary. However, overinclusiveness of a government's coercive power deprives some people of basic rights without proper justification. An example is a policy that imposes compulsory screening, isolation, or criminal penalties on groups *assumed* to be at a high risk of HIV infection. For instance, compulsory measures that apply to all homosexuals, commercial sex workers, IDUs, or persons from countries with high HIV infection rates stem from the erroneous belief that all members of the group engage in unprotected sex or needle sharing. Such policies are overbroad; while a few individuals may act in a risky way, most group members likely do not. To apply compulsory measures to persons who pose little or no risk of HIV transmission unjustifiably and inexcusably deprives them of autonomy, privacy, and liberty.

Some policies may be both under- and overinclusive. Consider a decision to criminally penalize sex workers but not their male agents (pimps) or clients (johns). This policy is suspiciously underinclusive because it selectively punishes a vulnerable population when two other groups actively participate in or profit from the risky behavior. The policy is also overinclusive because it applies to all sex workers, and some sex workers are not infected with HIV, inform their clients of the potential risks, and/or practice safer sex.

HIV/AIDS policies must be well targeted. To protect human rights, officials should evaluate whether the selected means achieve the public health objective and whether the policy includes appropriate groups.

Examine Each Policy for Possible Human Rights Burdens

Policymakers must balance the efficacy of an intervention against its impact on human rights. Even a well-focused and effective policy may unduly burden human rights. Identifying all potential infringements on human rights and evaluating those likely to occur can produce sound government action. For this step in policymaking, the core human rights principles described in Chapter 1 offer a reference, but are not exhaustive. Officials should enact policies that protect individuals' rights to security of person, equal treatment, liberty, privacy, family unity, free expression, free association, and other human rights.

Some policies so burden human rights that their public health benefit never outweighs such intrusions. That a policy improves public health does not automatically justify any possible means to achieve it. For instance, murder, genocide, torture, and inhuman and degrading treatment can never be justified. In contrast, minor infringements on privacy or autonomy may be justified where the public health interest is compelling. For example, requiring a population to be immunized by means of a safe and effective AIDS vaccine may undermine the right to security of person but may be justified by the substantial reduction in seroprevalence. A blinded survey of seroprevalence may not respect the principle of informed consent, but the epidemiological knowledge gained may outweigh the interference.

How does one measure the extent of a human rights burden? We suggest four factors: (1) the nature of the human right, (2) the invasiveness of the intervention, (3) the frequency and scope of the infringement, and (4) its duration. Policies that adversely affect fundamental individual rights, such as liberty and freedom of movement, are suspect. A decision to imprison, isolate, or otherwise restrict a person's liberty substantially impacts the person's life. In contrast, while reporting or notification requirements potentially infringe on privacy, this type of invasion is less grave than a deprivation of liberty.

The second factor examines the degree of intrusion on a particular right. Neither liberty nor privacy is absolute. All societies tolerate some incursions on these rights (e.g., limitations on individual liberty where it interferes with the fundamental rights of others, or disclosure of private information when its protection imminently endangers another person). However, burdens on either right may well outweigh a public health policy's potential benefits. For instance, a government's decision to record and grant public access to the names of persons infected with HIV deeply intrudes upon their privacy. Similarly, an initiative to prohibit all HIV-infected women from bearing children, based on the risk of HIV transmission, fundamentally burdens privacy in the context of reproductive decision-making.

A third question asks whether the deprivation applies to a few people or to an entire group or population. Levying criminal penalties against a person who intentionally stabs another with an HIV-contaminated needle or intentionally inflicts harm in a particularly egregious manner may be justified. However, a policy that quarantines a large population infected with HIV substantially burdens human rights. Imagine a government that intends to reduce the seroprevalence of HIV in its population by screening and isolating all persons who enter or return to the country. Although the government might argue that this policy would achieve a compelling public health objective, the gravity and scope of the human rights burdens would be prohibitive.

Fourth, the duration of a human rights burden may be instructive. Regarding quarantines, one might distinguish temporary deprivations of liberty from more extended ones. To isolate a person who is dually infected with HIV and tuberculosis (TB) during the active stage of tuberculosis is a necessary, short-term intervention; adequate TB treatment renders the person noncontagious for TB in a matter of weeks. However, isolating a person with HIV infection is almost always inappropriate; it would essentially confine a person indefinitely since the person remains "contagious" for life.

In sum, evaluating human rights burdens requires assessing *all* of the potential harms to persons or populations. Officials should ask: (1) What are the core human rights principles involved? (2) How powerfully does a policy invade the rights of a person or population? (3) How many people does the policy affect and how frequently? and (4) What is the duration of the human rights infringement? A sensitive understanding of what is at stake for the relevant population helps to ensure human rights protections.

Chapters 1 and 2 describe numerous international and regional human rights instruments and AIDS-related writings concerned with human rights. These documents can greatly assist in identifying human rights abuses. Human rights experts and nongovernmental organizations may be invaluable in assisting those trying to evaluate a policy's impact on human rights or attempting to enforce international protections. Establishing networks of experts in human rights and public health can facilitate constructive debate and may lead to greater respect for human rights in policy development, implementation, and enforcement.

Determine Whether the Policy Is the Least Restrictive Alternative That Can Achieve the Public Health Objective

The impact assessment suggests a balance between a policy's human rights burdens and its public health benefits. An approach that effectively achieves a compelling public health goal may sometimes warrant a derogation of human rights. In contrast, a dubious government interest deserves little weight in the balance. In addition to investigating the nature of the public health objective, officials should also evaluate the extent to which a policy deprives people of basic human rights. Broad or intrusive human rights violations are seldom, if ever, warranted, although minor interferences may be.

A vital step in the human rights impact assessment is the examination of alternative policies that burden human rights to a lesser extent. The principle of the least restrictive alternative recommends adopting the least intrusive policy that achieves the public health objective (Siracusa Principles, 1984). The human rights community should insist that, whenever possible, governments find less drastic alternatives that achieve the public health goal without unduly violating personal freedoms.

Public health officials sometimes misunderstand the principle of the least restrictive alternative. The principle does not require governments to adopt ineffective policies or to forego efficacious ones. Rather, the principle compels implementation of minimally burdensome programs that are equally or more effective in reducing the spread of HIV. On occasion, less intrusive alternatives are also less effective. But the human rights protections gained by demanding alternatives outweigh the exceptional cases.

To determine the least restrictive alternative, officials should consider noncoercive approaches first, and only if necessary gradually move to more intrusive measures. Examples of the former include counseling, education, treatment, and support services. If policymakers discover that these programs are insufficient, they may examine other minimally restrictive policies.

Governments are sometimes urged to implement restrictive measures to manage public health concerns. Policymakers must resist public pressure to blame foreigners, drug users, homosexuals, sex workers, or other disenfranchised populations. Officials should examine a policy's impact on public health and human rights by thoroughly considering less restrictive alternatives.

Although public health and human rights occasionally conflict, often the two are in harmony. Moreover, the two are frequently synergistic; protecting human rights encourages cooperation, a shared vision for safer behaviors, and promotion of public health.

If a Coercive Measure Is Truly the Most Effective, Least Restrictive Alternative, Base it on the "Significant Risk" Standard and Guarantee Fair Procedures

Determination of risk

After analyzing a range of policies, the health authority may conclude that a coercive approach is the most effective, least restrictive alternative. This requires an *individual determination* that the person poses a *significant risk* to the public.

The "significant risk" standard permits coercive measures only to avert likely harm to the health or safety of others. The determination of significant risk is a public health inquiry. The intent of human rights law is to replace decisions based on irrational fear, speculation, stereotypes, or pernicious mythologies with reasoned, scientifically valid judgments.

Significant risk must be determined on a case-by-case basis through fact-specific, individual inquiries. Blanket rules or generalizations about a class of persons with HIV infection do not suffice. The risk must be "significant," not merely speculative or remote. For example, theoretically, a person could transmit HIV by biting, spitting, or splattering blood, but the actual risk is extremely low (approaching zero). Likewise, an HIV-infected health care professional who does not perform deeply invasive procedures is highly unlikely to transmit HIV to a patient. Present knowledge does not support screening or excluding that person from the health care profession because, lacking a real and substantial possibility of HIV transmission, such policies do not meet the significant risk test.

Public health interventions should focus on *modes of transmission* supported by epidemiological studies. Current information holds that sexual intercourse and sharing contaminated drug injection equipment constitute "significant risks." Biting, spitting, or rough play in schools or sports, however, do not meet this test and cannot support compulsory screening, exclusion, or isolation. Similarly, the *possibility* that food service workers may bleed into food or that airline pilots might suddenly experience AIDS dementia is so low that it does not justify depriving a class of professionals of their rights and livelihood.

The significant risk requirement maintains that although HIV infection can be fatal, restrictions are unjustifiable unless based upon a reasonable probability of transmission. For instance, some parents wonder why school officials exclude from classes children infested with head lice but not those infected with HIV. The significant risk standard is met in the former case because a high probability exists that other children will contract lice; in contrast, the risk of contracting HIV in a school setting is extremely remote.

Fair procedures

International human rights standards require that governments provide a fair public hearing before depriving persons of liberty, the right to travel, or other fundamental rights (see, e.g., Art. 8 and 10 of the Universal Declaration of Human Rights and Art. 5 of the European Convention of Human Rights). That a public health intervention is not intended to be punitive does not detract from the fact that it robs a person of liberty. In this respect, the public health justifications resemble those in the mental health context. Specifically, the United Nations Declaration on the Rights of Persons with Mental Illness (1991a) requires procedural safeguards known as "due process" in North America and "natural justice" in many other areas of the world. As in the mental health setting, public health policies that deprive people of liberty to protect the public must guarantee procedural justice.

As construed by the European Court of Human Rights, the natural justice principle requires that an objective decisionmaker who is separate from the executive branch and the parties to the case hold a hearing (*X v. United Kingdom*, 1981; *Winterwerp v. The Netherlands*, 1979; *Van der Leer v. The Netherlands*, 1990). An independent court or tribunal must adjudicate the dispute. The person whose liberty is threatened is entitled to advance notice, representation, and an opportunity to present evidence.

Procedural safeguards are not merely formalistic. Their aim is to ensure accurate fact-finding and greater equity and fairness to individuals who face a loss of liberty. In addition, hearings give public health officials the opportunity to review their approach to controlling the AIDS epidemic and its practical and personal impact.

A government that deprives an individual of liberty or other rights must grant him a fair and public hearing and demonstrate that he poses a significant risk to the public. These substantive and procedural requirements help ensure that governments demonstrate a genuine need to initiate compulsory measures to protect the community and preserve individual justice.

CONCLUSION

By addressing human rights, governments are likely to enhance public health. Public health programs that respect human rights will encourage individuals and communities to trust and cooperate with public health authorities. Promotion of human rights, particularly among previously disenfranchised groups, enables them to protect their own health. Finally, health is a basic human right, related to and dependent on many other human rights (see Chapters 1 [substantive rights] and 4 [policies affecting those rights]). Therefore, government efforts to promote the right to health necessarily implicate a broad range of human rights. The Human Rights Impact Assessment assists government officials in achieving the best possible public health outcomes that simultaneously protect and promote human rights.

4

AIDS Policies and Practices: Integrating Public Health and Human Rights

For far too long, public health practitioners have developed policies as if the health of populations were distinct from human rights. Viewing public health and human rights as separate, or even antagonistic, is misguided and harmful to public health practice. Respect for the rights of human beings is a fundamental condition for health. Public health, then, needs to forge a conceptual and practical link with the social justice inherent in human rights.

This chapter examines traditional AIDS policies in both developing and more developed countries. Using the Human Rights Impact Assessment (see Chapter 3) public health and human rights imperatives are integrated into policymaking.

PREVENTION AND EDUCATION

Introduction

The modern history of public health shows that biomedical interventions are rarely sufficient to bring disease epidemics under control (Brandt, 1987). The most effective vaccines and medical treatments cannot fully contain disease epidemics, especially among very young or very old people and those living in poverty. Biomedical interventions are most unrealistic in less developed countries that lack adequate resources to buy or distribute the technology. For example, many countries continue to experience epidemics of sexually transmitted diseases, hepatitis, and tuberculosis, despite scientific achievements in treating or preventing these diseases through immunization. For HIV, no vaccine has yet proved safe and effective and biomedical treatments are only effective in delaying the onset of AIDS and preventing opportunistic infections. Zidovudine (AZT) may be effective in reducing the risk of perinatal transmission (from approximately twenty-five to eight percent); combination therapy with antiretroviral drugs may suppress the virus below levels of detection in infected adults: These are the first rays of hope for medical interventions (Centers for Disease Control and Prevention, 1994; Hammer, 1996; Ho, 1996). However, even the most basic antiviral medications and drugs designed to prevent opportunistic infections are largely unavailable in developing countries.

Given the limited role of biomedical interventions, particularly among poorer populations, prevention and education strategies offer the best possibility to stop the spread of HIV infection. An urgent need exists in all parts of the world for carefully designed prevention and education programs.

Goals of Prevention and Education

The goals of prevention and education programs are (1) to prevent new HIV infections by informing people about behaviors that transmit infection and by providing culturally and personally relevant means to alter behavior; (2) to improve the quality of life of individuals with HIV infection through early diagnosis, counseling, humane treatment, and continuing care and support; (3) to provide information, advocacy, and resources to empower vulnerable people and communities to fight discrimination and exploitation; and (4) to reduce discrimination by eliminating ignorance, stereotypes, and irrational fear of persons with HIV infection or AIDS (United States National Commission on AIDS, 1991).

Prevention strategies that provide clear and personally relevant information and counseling promote human rights and public health. Applying the Human Rights Impact Assessment, we find (1) that the public health objective of health education is compelling; (2) that substantial empirical data support the efficacy of well-targeted prevention strategies; (3) that such a program targets persons who are at risk of contracting or transmitting infection; and (4) that the program is noncoercive in that it poses no demonstrable public health burdens. Efforts to replace fears and prejudices with accurate information promote human rights and public health by reducing the discrimination faced by traditionally disfavored groups who also tend to experience HIV-related discrimination.

Education and Prevention Efforts and Human Rights Burdens

Human rights violations occur when states *fail* to provide adequate AIDS education. The Universal Declaration of Human Rights (Art. 26.2) and the International Covenant on Economic, Social and Cultural Rights (Art. 13.2[a]) guarantee all persons a right to education. Education must promote understanding and tolerance (UDHR, Art. 26.2; ICESCR, Art. 13.1) as well as the full development of the human personality. The Universal Declaration of Human Rights (Art. 19) and International Covenant of Civil and Political Rights (Art. 19) provide the right to free expression, including the right to seek, receive, and impart information of all kinds, either orally, in writing, in the form of art, or through any other medium (see Chapter 1: Freedom of Opinion and Expression). The government's failure to adequately inform the public about HIV violates the state's duty to educate. Censoring the exchange of HIV/AIDS information infringes on the right to the free flow of information. A serious lack of education or free exchange of information can impede citizens' ability to protect their health and their lives.

Ironically, even the discovery of a biomedical intervention with substantial potential to prevent HIV infection, such as zidovudine treatment during pregnancy to reduce the risk of perinatal transmission, can pose human rights problems. Where health care providers or public officials know of the intervention but do not inform pregnant women of its efficacy, they fail to arm women with the information necessary to protect themselves and their children (see Chapter 1: The Right to Education). Where zidovudine (or other effective drugs for treatment and prophylaxis of opportunistic infections) is unavailable, women have a human rights claim to benefit from scientific advances, as well as an ethical claim for equitable distribution of effective pharmaceuticals (see Chapter 1: The Right to Share in the Benefits of Scientific and Technological Progress). Even where zidovudine is available and women are informed of its potential efficacy, however, human rights issues remain. Discovery of an effective intervention may provoke calls for mandatory HIV testing of all pregnant women and mandatory treatment of infected women (Bayer, 1994). If implemented, such policies would substantially burden women's fundamental rights to security of person and privacy, among others (see this chapter, *Epidemiological Surveillance and Disease Control*).

Additionally, prevention strategies involving access to health information may threaten human rights in several ways, including (1) government failure to ensure full and objective information necessary to protect health, (2) government control or censorship of educational messages, and (3) nongovernmental institutional (e.g., church or family) control or censorship of educational messages.

Failure of government to ensure full and objective information

The scientific community knows a great deal about how HIV is transmitted and what behavioral changes slow its spread. In a relatively short time, epidemiological research has revealed more about HIV than any other human retrovirus. Studies show rapid and profound, but predictably insufficient, behavioral changes in certain populations that participate in comprehensive health education programs (e.g., homosexual men, injecting drug users, and commercial sex workers) (Auerbach, Wypijewska, et al., 1994; Higgins, Galavotti, et al., 1991; Becker, Joseph, 1988). Some communities have significantly reduced risky behavior, evidenced by marked declines in new infection rates. Programs that promote behavioral changes have the best chance of long-lasting success if they also address the deeper problems that leave some citizens more vulnerable than others to HIV infection (e.g., drug addiction, sexual exploitation, and domestic violence). Research suggests that people have the capacity to alter behavior that is deeply entrenched or even physically addictive (Normand, Vlahov, et al., 1995; Groseclose, Weinstein, et al., 1995; Paone, Des Jarlais, et al., 1994; Watters, 1994).

Effective prevention programs are not quick fixes that can be applied once to a target population with lasting effects (Auerbach, Wypijewska, et al., 1994). Most studies that have documented long-term behavior change have involved ongoing, periodic, or repeated counseling, often of couples or very small groups, to promote safer sexual behavior (De Vincenzi, 1994; Padian, O'Brien, et al., 1993). For example, one study found only limited evidence of short-term behavior change among college students who received written information, a didactic lecture, and small group discussion (Turner, Korpita, et al., 1993).

States should design educational messages and supply resources to achieve the public health objective. Efforts must reach persons at every level of society, including the general public, schoolchildren, and groups particularly at risk. States should present clear and objective health information. More importantly, communities and individuals must understand and apply norms of safer behavior. Successful education efforts begin with appreciation for the worth and uniqueness of the individual and community. Educational messages must be linguistically, culturally, and personally responsive to the persons who receive them. This helps to promote behavioral change, cultural respect, and social acceptance (Burris, 1992).

Educational efforts tend to fail unless individuals have the *means* with which to follow public health advice (Des Jarlais, Friedman, 1988). Persons who engage in unprotected sex or share injection equipment will not simply stop because messages advocate abstinence. They require access to the means to do so. Accordingly, condoms, sterile injection equipment, and other tools are necessary to obtain the desired health benefits (see also in this chapter, Harm Reduction Strategies; Personal Control Measures).

Even with culturally appropriate information and means, many people need assistance to modify their behavior. Some individuals in society lack the ability to protect themselves and improve their well-being. For example, monogamous women in some parts of the world contract HIV infection because they cannot influence their partners' extramarital sexual behavior, and they lack the power to refuse sex or to insist that their partners use condoms (Reid, 1990). Cultural, economic, and political forces condone extramarital sexual activity by men while reinforcing women's subordination. Women who question their partners' extramarital sexual activity or request that their partners use a condom may face physical and psychological abuse, deprivation, or personal and economic abandonment (United Nations, 1991).

The right to education is crucial in the context of public health and the HIV/AIDS pandemic. Knowledge enables people to protect themselves and others. To ensure rights to education and health, governments must impart information, supply appropriate means, and reduce societal exploitation and powerlessness. Government-sponsored AIDS education occupies the front line of defense against harm to public health and human rights.

Control or censorship of educational messages by government

Unfortunately, some governments have done more to limit AIDS education than to facilitate it. State interference assumes many forms—ranging from failing to fund education adequately to censoring educational messages. Restrictive policies may interfere with the rights to free expression, information, and education by limiting data collection and dissemination, barring syringe or condom distribution programs, or regulating the instructional content concerning sexual activity and drug use. A government may offer religious or moral reasons to justify such interferences, believing that such information encourages sex or drug use. Frank information about these issues potentially offends some parts of the community. But selectively withholding explicit information may deprive persons of information that they need to protect their health and lives. Moreover, a considerable amount of research fails to establish that educating people about AIDS or distributing clean needles or condoms encourages dangerous sexual behavior or drug use (Normand, Vlahov, et al., 1995; Lurie, Reingold, et al., 1993; Des Jarlais, Friedman, 1988).

When government actively censors or impedes the free flow of AIDS information, it does not merely interfere with the "positive" rights to education, health, and life. It also violates the "negative" right to free expression and information (see Chapter 1: Freedom of Opinion and Expression). This includes the right of scientists, health care workers, advocates, and individuals to exchange freely current information on AIDS prevention and treatment. It also includes the public's right, with few exceptions, to receive that information uncensored. The international human rights framework recognizes the government's right to restrict the exchange of information under certain circumstances, as where necessary to protect the public order, public health, or morals (ICCPR, Art. 19.3[b]). In most cases, policymakers would have difficulty justifying restrictions of HIV prevention information and education on the grounds of protecting the public order, public health, or morals. In this context, censorship is more likely to harm the public health than to protect it.

A government's first responsibility in addressing AIDS should be to promote public health and to protect human rights. This requires government to open the channels of communication. States should do everything within their power to ensure public understanding of modes of HIV transmission and to provide assistance with behavioral changes that protect against disease.

Control or censorship of educational messages by private institutions and persons

Families and religious, spiritual, and community leaders lack the formal powers of government to control or censor health information. Yet their impact on education, values, and lifestyles can be just as potent. A parent may strongly object to her child attending

AIDS education classes in school. A religious or community leader may oppose condom advertisements in public places. Parents, religious, and community leaders may argue that AIDS education and prevention programs infringe on their religious beliefs and their right to freely choose the religious and moral education of their children. Thus the human rights of some individuals may directly conflict with the rights of others. Private activities that undermine AIDS education programs pose fundamental problem for the public health and human rights communities. Although human rights offers no easy solutions, the following approach may facilitate a resolution that is acceptable to all.

Officials need to enlist the support of parents and church or community leaders in health education programs. Human rights advocates understand that principles of family unity demand respect for parental decisions; indeed, Article 26.3 of the Universal Declaration acknowledges parents' right to choose their children's education (see also ICESCR, Art. 13.3). Furthermore, principles of free expression protect *all* speech. Therefore, human rights and public health officials need to communicate with parents and religious, spiritual, and community leaders to forge mutual understandings. To accommodate moral and public health concerns, prevention policies can include discussions of abstinence or other ethical values shared by the community.

Where accommodation of effective information and community values is impossible public health personnel face a dilemma. International human rights law, as well as most domestic governments' policies, imposes on public health officials the duty to protect the health of individuals and the community. Where full and frank information on HIV will save lives, public health workers may feel obligated to disseminate that information even if it offends community standards. In each case, however, public health personnel should weigh the possible negative consequences of their acts against the potential benefits. If the program alienates the community or drastically reduces cooperation with other effective public health measures to control HIV and other diseases, the potential harm may outweigh the program's benefits (see Chapter 1: When Rights Conflict).

Conclusion

The rights to education, health, and life create corresponding duties for government to educate the community. The rights to free expression and the free exchange of information protect individuals and public health advocates who disseminate information to communities and across borders. Education leads to knowledge, power, and opportunity: the knowledge of behaviors that cause ill-health and disease, the power to make changes to preserve health and life, and the opportunity to be free from stigma and discrimination.

Nicholas Freudenberg (1990) has noted:

> The reality is that a world without AIDS, or a world with this epidemic under control, will look very different. It will be a world where everyone is entitled to comprehensive educa

tion about sexuality, drugs, and health; a world where basic health care is a right; a world where gay men, lesbians, women and people of color are not discriminated against; a world where no one has to die on the streets because there is no home for them.

Effective education rests upon the free exchange of information and is part of a web of human and social services. Education breeds tolerance for differences and respect for human dignity. It indeed can help make our world look very different.

ANTIDISCRIMINATION POLICIES

Introduction

A series of reports from Luis Varela Quiros (United Nations, 1991, 1992, 1993), United Nations Special Rapporteur to the Sub-Commission on the Prevention of Discrimination and Protection of Minorities, reveals that discrimination against persons with HIV infection or AIDS remains widespread and occurs at all levels of society, including government, public and private institutions, and among individuals and communities. Discriminatory conduct is directed at those with HIV infection or AIDS, as well as their families, friends, and caregivers. The HIV/AIDS pandemic has intensified preexisting prejudices against communities associated with the disease.

International health and human rights organizations have resoundingly condemned discrimination against persons with HIV infection or AIDS. Such discrimination is based on status and is prohibited under international human rights provisions (see Chapter 1: Nondiscrimination).

By the end of the first decade of the HIV/AIDS pandemic (1981–1991), 104 countries had adopted HIV/AIDS-related legislation (Tomasevski, Gruskin, et al., 1992; World Health Organization, 1993a). Some legislation protects the rights of persons infected with HIV or strengthens HIV/AIDS education efforts. Many national AIDS programs assert a policy of nondiscrimination related to AIDS. As of 1995, however, a report by the United Nations Secretary-General concluded that few countries had taken explicit steps to enact and implement antidiscrimination provisions with the force of law (United Nations, 1995c). Many laws instead foster stigmatization, harassment, or discrimination against population groups or individuals associated with the pandemic. These laws include mandatory screening of homosexuals, sex workers, injection drug users, foreigners, or other perceived "risk groups"; prohibition of HIV-infected persons from certain professions; isolation, detention, compulsory treatment, or medical examination of persons with HIV infection; limitations on international travel by requiring HIV testing for entry into certain countries; classification of HIV/AIDS as a special or dangerous disease requiring differential treatment by medical personnel; and the requirement that AIDS be listed on death certificates. Criminal sanctions for homosexuality, prostitution, and injection drug use have contributed to stigmatization, increased the spread of HIV, and hindered prevention efforts (United Nations, 1992).

The Public Health Purpose

Public health experts have long maintained that no public health rationale justifies restricting the rights and liberties of people solely because they have HIV infection or AIDS (World Health Organization, 1987a; World Summit of Ministers of Health, 1988; World Health Assembly, Forty-first, 1988; World Health Assembly, Forty-fifth, 1992). Likewise, discrimination based on HIV status is unjustified in the areas of housing, employment, and education (World Health Organization, 1989b).

In contrast, the public health purpose for adopting formal antidiscrimination laws and policies is compelling. Discriminatory policies and practices can endanger the public health by forcing those who are infected to "go underground" to avoid detection. Policies which protect individuals from discrimination may encourage them to seek counseling, testing, and education as well as increase their access to health care and other social services (see also this chapter, Epidemiological Surveillance and Disease Control; The Health Care System).

Well-designed antidiscrimination provisions are well targeted and aim to protect people vulnerable to discrimination. Such provisions do not permit the state to infringe on an individual's rights but rather protect him from public and private abuses. Consequently, their burdens on human rights should be minimal.

Sources and Impact of Discrimination

Discriminatory policies, programs, or actions are often based on irrational fears, ignorance, or misconceptions about people with HIV/AIDS or on underlying prejudices against particular racial, ethnic, or other minorities. The primary misconception about HIV is that it can be spread through casual contact. This belief has led to misguided responses—excluding children from schools, dismissing employees from jobs, evicting families from housing, excluding health care professionals from practice, and others—when little or no risk of infection exists.

Throughout the world, the interrelationship between racism and AIDS discrimination has been profound (Sabatier, 1988). Sometimes racism is overt, as in efforts to "blame" one race or an entire country or continent for "starting" the pandemic. More subtle variations involve the inclusion of ethnic or racial groups among "risk groups" regardless of individual behavior, or the testing of students or workers from certain parts of the world but not others. Popular suspicion of racist motives runs so deep that some individuals believe that AIDS is a form of genocide against their race or ethnic group (Dalton, 1989).

Stigmatization of persons with HIV infection or AIDS can lead to discriminatory acts within communities and families. Persons with HIV/AIDS have eloquently described the dehumanization and isolation they have felt when families or communities shun them, consigning them to virtual "civil death" (Daniel, 1992). In many regions, the death from

AIDS of many men and women in their prime childrearing years has rapidly increased the number of orphans (Preble, 1990; Michaels, Levine, 1992; Caldwell, Fleming, et al., 1992). In other countries, babies known to have or suspected of having HIV infection are abandoned. In addition to the difficulty of finding homes for new orphans, families and communities in both developed and developing countries are hesitant to adopt children who have been orphaned or abandoned due to AIDS (see Chapter 1: The Right to Marry and Found a Family).

One of the tragic consequences of discrimination is that it deeply impacts vulnerable groups. Relatively powerless persons, including women, men who have sex with men, injection drug users, and poor and homeless people, are at greater risk of HIV infection because of their inability to protect themselves. HIV infection compounds their vulnerability to invidious discrimination and ill-treatment (United Nations 1995a–c, 1989f; Paris Declaration on Women, Children and AIDS, 1989). For example, women are often discriminated against in education, training, and employment, which leads them to depend socially and economically on men. Once dependent on a particular relationship, some women may have difficulty protecting themselves from HIV infection. They may not be able to insist that their sexual partner use a condom during intercourse for fear of verbal or physical abuse or abandonment (Worth, 1989). Once infected, women may be rejected by their families, stigmatized within their communities, blamed for their own infection and that of their partners or children, and physically abused by their sexual partners (Hamblin, Reid, 1991; North, Rothenberg, 1993).

Antidiscrimination Legislation

To mitigate discrimination requires developing a more supportive environment for persons with HIV infection or AIDS. As a first step, states should review existing laws and practices and repeal those that discriminate or encourage discrimination against persons with HIV. The United Nations Secretary-General has called upon member states to review their AIDS policies for evidence of discrimination and other human rights abuses, to ensure full enjoyment of civil, political, economic, social, and cultural rights by persons with HIV, and to provide legal redress for persons who experience HIV-related discrimination (United Nations, 1995c, 1996a).

Policymakers differ on the usefulness of antidiscrimination legislation in protecting the rights of persons with HIV/AIDS. Some argue that national antidiscrimination legislation should be introduced immediately to create a structure to protect persons with HIV/AIDS. Others who also oppose HIV-related discrimination suggest that litigation may not provide relief for persons with HIV/AIDS due to the delay, stress, and expense of litigation. Some doubt whether many jurisdictions will enforce laws that are contrary to long-standing practices and existing discriminatory policies and programs. The United Nations Special Rapporteur, however, notes that some states that have adopted antidiscrimination polices indicate that those policies can provide an effective framework for educating employers and others to avoid discrimination (United Nations, 1992). Thus, antidiscrimination laws provide education and normative examples for all members of society regarding HIV infection and AIDS, act as a deterrent to future discrimination, and offer relief for persons unjustifiably denied rights or benefits.

The concluding statement of a Pan-European Consultation on HIV/AIDS recommended that states consider introducing legislation to protect individuals from HIV-related discrimination in employment, education, travel, access to social services, and health care (World Health Organization, 1991). As of mid-1991, at least fourteen countries had adopted national AIDS antidiscrimination legislation (Curran, Gostin, et al., 1991).

Antidiscrimination legislation may focus exclusively on persons with HIV infection or AIDS or may apply to all persons with disabilities. Australia provides a potentially effective model that specifically bars discrimination against persons with HIV infection or AIDS (Department of Health, Housing and Community Services, 1992). The Americans with Disabilities Act (ADA), implemented in the United States in 1992, illustrates a more generic approach to antidiscrimination (Gostin, 1992a). The ADA prohibits discrimination against all persons with disabilities including those with serious physical or mental illnesses, tuberculosis, cancer, or heart disease. The Act protects HIV-infected individuals at all stages, from asymptomatic infection to active disease. It also protects persons who are not infected, but are *perceived* to be so. The Act prohibits discrimination in employment, government services, telecommunications, and transportation in both the public and private sectors (Americans with Disabilities Act, 1990).

An antidiscrimination law alone may not change people's *beliefs* about persons with HIV infection or AIDS, but it can change the way people *behave*. Societies have a moral obligation to ensure respect and equal treatment in all aspects of life for persons with disabilities—including HIV-positive individuals. Persons with disabilities have more than their own physical handicaps with which to contend. They must withstand the burden of myths, fears, and stereotypes. All individuals can contribute to their families, employers, and communities if given a full and equal opportunity to do so.

EPIDEMIOLOGICAL SURVEILLANCE AND DISEASE CONTROL

Introduction

In addition to education and prevention programs, states should conduct epidemiological surveillance and disease control efforts as part of a comprehensive defense against AIDS. A number of policies fit within this category; this section discusses testing and screening, reporting and notification of HIV-antibody test results for epidemiological purposes, and partner notification.

Testing and Screening

The test for HIV antibodies, developed in 1985, is an important technological tool for HIV prevention and treatment. Yet states may misuse test results in ways that burden human rights and impede efforts to control the spread of infection.

Prior to implementing a screening program, states must consider the matter of technical accuracy (Brandt, Cleary, et al., 1990, p. 126). Policymakers should determine which combination of tests best achieves the goal of a particular program. Specifically, they should recognize the potential for a high proportion of false positives in populations with very low seroprevalence; the potential for false negatives among persons recently infected but not yet seroconverted; human error in interpreting test results; and the difficulty of maintaining high technical standards when performing numerous tests.

The human rights impact assessment requires a determination of whether a particular screening program serves a compelling public health purpose, whether it burdens human rights, and, if so, whether an alternative minimizes such burdens while achieving equally well the public health goal.

The human rights burdens from HIV testing programs vary depending on program design and implementation. To evaluate the human rights impact, public officials should consider whether the testing is voluntary; whether informed consent is sought; whether consent is coupled with pre- and post-test counseling; whether confidential information is protected; and whether test results are used to exclude persons from benefits or services. Additionally, officials should examine screening policies and programs for discriminatory motives or effects.

Voluntariness

Testing programs are most beneficial when they are voluntary. In 1992, a consultation of World Health Organization experts concluded, "There are no benefits either to the individual or for public health arising from testing without informed consent that cannot be achieved by less intrusive means, such as voluntary testing and counseling" (1992h).

States should require informed consent and should provide pre- and post-test counseling. Informed consent requires that a patient know the test's nature, purpose, and risks, be competent to understand and evaluate the information supplied, and voluntarily agree, without coercion, to the test. This approach respects both the ethical principle of patient autonomy and the human rights goal of individual autonomy and security of person (see Chapter 1: Right to Security). In addition, voluntary testing with counseling and informed consent can facilitate behavior modification through knowledge of the risks and benefits of different behaviors. Early detection of HIV infection can benefit the individual, through early treatment, prophylaxis of opportunistic infections, and screening for tuberculosis (Fischl, Richman, et al., 1987; Sande, Carpenter, et al., 1993).

Perhaps the most compelling rationale for widespread population screening is that the counseling that may accompany it encourages safer behavior. Voluntary testing alone is unlikely to effect long-lasting behavioral change. Professional counseling before and after the test creates a supportive climate in which individuals are more likely to alter their conduct prudently, regardless of test results (Auerbach, Wypijewska, et al., 1994). In contrast, compulsory testing reduces the likelihood that a person will either cooperate or change behavior. Moreover, it may drive people at risk away from the health care system due to fear that they will be tested against their will (Field, 1990). The testing process should embrace a persuasive rather than a coercive approach. The World Health Organization and most other professional bodies strongly support voluntary testing, accompanied by appropriate counseling, to reduce the spread of HIV infection (World Health Organization, 1992h, 1988d; Centers for Disease Control and Prevention, 1993b, 1987).

Therapeutic innovations for persons with HIV infection further support voluntary testing, provided those persons infected are reasonably likely to receive treatment. AZT and other retroviral drugs can slow the course of HIV disease and perhaps delay the onset of AIDS (Fischl, Richman, et al., 1987). Many developed countries use effective prophylaxis for pneumocystis carinii pneumonia (PCP), TB, and other opportunistic infections associated with HIV disease (Centers for Disease Control and Prevention, 1995a,b). Unfortunately, most of the world's individuals infected with HIV live in countries where retroviral medications and prophylaxis are not available. Likewise, poor people in many developed countries have limited access to costly treatments.

Substantial inequalities in access to treatment raise human rights concerns (e.g., the rights of poorer persons and countries to share in the benefits of science and technology, the right to health, and the right to life) (see Chapter 1: The Right to Life; The Right to Health; The Right to Share in the Benefits of Scientific and Technological Progress). States that establish screening programs to encourage early diagnosis and treatment should ensure that people actually receive the explicitly or implicitly promised benefits. Even where treatment is available, however, the potential benefit to the individual does not justify compulsory testing. Many civil- and common-law countries prohibit treatment without consent, even when treatment offers benefits. The right to security of person allows each individual to decide for him- or herself whether to be tested and treated.

The availability of a new technology or treatment may also spur calls for mandatory testing. Since the potential efficacy of zidovudine in reducing perinatal transmission was reported, some commentators and policymakers have proposed mandatory testing of pregnant women (American Medical Association, 1996; Altman, 1994; Bayer, 1994). Such testing, however, would substantially burden women's security of person and privacy. Intensive education and voluntary testing of pregnant women at risk of HIV infection would burden women's human rights much less. Moreover, since zidovudine treatment currently involves an extended period of treatment before, during, and after birth, mandatory testing could decrease the program's effectiveness if it discourages cooperation and trust between pregnant women and health care providers or causes women to avoid pre- or postnatal care (Bayer, 1994; Minkoff, Willoughby, 1995). For these reasons, the U.S. Centers for Disease Control recommends that all testing of pregnant women and infants be voluntary and that women who refuse testing should not be denied care, reported to child protective services, or discriminated against in any other way (Centers for Disease Control and Prevention, 1995c).

Public health rationales for screening include the need to assess accurately the seroprevalence in a population, prevent the spread of HIV through tainted blood donations, and prevent occupational exposures to HIV. Widespread screening, however, is an imperfect tool for epidemiological assessment because of the biases involved in a self-selected population. Moreover, because screening involves the systematic collection of intimate health information, it risks breaches of confidentiality.

Researchers have used "unlinked anonymous [or blinded] screening" (UAS) as a method of epidemiological surveillance that is both more reliable and less invasive of human rights. Where blood has been withdrawn for another purpose (such as routine serologic testing prior to hospital admission or at birth), researchers may test excess blood for evidence of HIV infection. To protect confidentiality and avoid the need for consent, all personal identifying information is removed prior to the test. The results of UAS are used for epidemiological purposes only.

Unlinked anonymous screening may provide a reliable estimate of the seroprevalence in limited groups (e.g., patients in hospitals, prenatal clinics, or sexually transmitted disease or drug addiction treatment centers). The method, however, harbors drawbacks. First, the accuracy of the results is limited to each group; researchers can seldom draw reliable generalizations from this data to the broader population. Second, UAS raises ethical questions. The design of screening programs usually makes it impossible to inform those persons who test positive for HIV. Commentators in some countries have questioned whether sufficient public health justification exists where patients are denied the right to know personal medical information, and health care providers have a duty to inform patients and, potentially, third parties at risk of infection (Bayer, Lumey, et al., 1991; Kastelein, Legemaate, et al., 1990; Bauder, 1994). One possible compromise is to match a patient and his test by code so that upon request he could learn his serostatus. Alternatively, UAS programs could include information on where to receive a linked test conveniently and free of charge. Despite the inherent limitations of the data and the risk that some individuals will be denied medical information about themselves, the ethical foundations for blinded screening have been widely accepted by ethicists and public health organizations (Bayer, 1995; World Health Organization, 1989f).

The use of screening or testing to prevent HIV transmission through contaminated blood or tissue and within the medical workplace is examined in more detail elsewhere (see this chapter, The Health Care System).

Confidentiality

Policymakers should design testing and screening programs that protect against breaches of confidentiality. Policies may protect confidentiality by purposefully eliminating identifying information. Two examples are anonymous testing programs, where the person taking the HIV antibody test is known only by a number, and UAS, where blood samples are separated from all personal identifiers. Policymakers may also protect confidentiality by implementing rigorous safeguards, fortified by law to prevent unauthorized disclosures.

Screening programs that collect information on intimate behaviors possess the potential for privacy violations and discrimination. For example, blood banks routinely ask if persons have engaged in high-risk activities. Special protections for HIV-related data need to accompany such programs. Policies that allow authorities to collect and share personally identifiable data pose the greatest risks of confidentiality breaches and subsequent discrimination against persons tested. Precisely these kinds of programs can discourage participation by persons who fear they are infected.

Discrimination

Invidious motives may influence targeted screening programs, since HIV infection is often associated with racial, ethnic, or sexual minorities, the poor, and other marginalized groups. In design or implementation, programs may discriminate against specific communities. Furthermore, the results of screening may lead to discrimination in housing, education, insurance, and access to medical care or to stigmatization by families or communities (see Chapter 1: Nondiscrimination; The Right to Marry and Found a Family).

Exclusion from benefits, privileges, or services

Testing programs should aim to inform persons at risk of HIV infection of their serological status and to provide an opportunity for counseling, education, and early treatment. Unfortunately, some governments use testing to exclude people from benefits and services (e.g,, testing persons to deprive them of the right to travel or testing immigrants to exclude them from services). Similarly, states may use premarital screening to discourage or prohibit marriage; may test prisoners or other institutionalized populations to segregate those infected with HIV; and may test accused criminals to obtain more punitive sentences.

To employ screening programs to disadvantage persons, to impose social control, or to punish constitutes a perversion of scientific and public health tools. At the very least, screening programs that exclude persons from benefits and services must be rigorously scrutinized for additional human rights violations such as the right to family life (e.g., premarital or prenatal screening), the right to liberty (e.g., isolation or quarantine), and the right to education or to work (e.g., excluding HIV-infected children from school or adults from certain occupations).

Reporting

AIDS was first described from reports and investigations of unusual clusters of opportunistic infections and rare cancers (Centers for Disease Control and Prevention, 1981; Masur, Michelis, et al., 1981). Based on this, researchers were able, relatively rapidly, to determine the probable modes of transmission (Francis, Curran, et al., 1983) and to isolate the causative agent, HIV. Sensitive, accurate, timely surveillance and reporting, and investigation of unusual or unexplained illnesses and deaths together constitute one of the primary strategies proposed by the Institute of Medicine (1992) and the U.S. Centers for Disease Control (1994) to combat the threat of other emerging and reemerging infectious diseases.

HIV/AIDS reporting programs usually require compliance by physicians, laboratories, or hospitals. Some countries, such as the Netherlands, maintain an entirely voluntary system (Bayer, Lumey, et al., 1991).

In many countries, notifying or reporting AIDS cases or HIV-positive test results to a central authority (local, state, provincial, or national) is a core part of the epidemiological surveillance system (Curran, Gostin, et al., 1991). As with reporting systems for any disease, those for HIV/AIDS vary greatly in efficiency and accuracy. The program's merit depends upon who notifies the authority, how quickly, how much paperwork is involved, and how data are used, stored, and made available.

Reporting AIDS cases alone underestimates the severity of the epidemic because the number of HIV-infected persons who will eventually develop clinical AIDS always far exceeds the number of AIDS cases. This is particularly true for countries in the early stages of the epidemic. For example, in Southeast Asia in 1992, an estimated 100,000 people had AIDS, while an estimated 800,000 were infected with HIV (Mann, Tarantola, et al., 1992). Reporting HIV infection figures most accurately reflects the epidemic's intensity in a given population. Such reporting, however, does not produce entirely reliable seroprevalence estimates due to selection bias in who is tested.

Reports of AIDS cases may underestimate the epidemic's severity due to medical personnel's failure to diagnose the disease, lack of functioning reporting systems, overburdened health care facilities, or fear and stigma. Underdiagnosis and subsequent underreporting are especially likely to occur when clinicians lack experience with AIDS, when relative morbidity and mortality are high, and when laboratory confirmation of cause of death is unusual.

To illustrate, in 1995, official reports of AIDS cases in India topped 2,000. Researchers currently estimate that actually tens of thousands of persons have AIDS, and one to two million Indians are likely to be currently infected with HIV (Shreedhar, 1995).

Reporting programs raise human rights concerns primarily for breaches of confidentiality. Individuals and advocates should investigate whether the reporting is anonymous or identifiable, whether the data are shared and with whom, how the data are used, whether special confidentiality protections exist, and whether legal safeguards protect against and punish unauthorized disclosures (Gostin, Lazzarini, et al., 1996a; Tomasevski, Gruskin, et al., 1992). States that require the reporting of AIDS or HIV infection may protect confidentiality by either collecting only anonymous information or by protecting information through "the strictest compliance with medical confidentiality—that is, it would only be released either anonymously, or with the express and informed consent of the person to whom it related" (United Nations Centre for Human Rights, 1989b).

Partner Notification

The traditional public health approach to control sexually transmitted and communicable diseases has often included identifying, examining, testing, and treating people who may have come into contact with index (known) cases. In regard to HIV/AIDS, where local law permits partner notification, public health professionals usually hold confidential discussions with infected persons about their past and current sexual or needle-sharing partners. The public health workers contact persons who may have been exposed to HIV and offer them education, counseling, and testing. The program design usually protects the identity of the possible source of infection and thus helps to ensure confidentiality. A breach of confidentiality may result, however, where the partner of the index case has had but a few sexual or needle-sharing partners.

Views differ regarding the appropriate design of partner notification programs for HIV/AIDS. One perspective favors the traditional public health approach described which protects the index case's identity. A second approach holds that health care professionals have a duty to inform partners of the risk of infection, including the identity of the possible source (for a detailed discussion of disclosure of HIV-related information to third parties, see Chapter 1: Privacy).

The public health benefits of partner notification programs depend on several factors: the seroprevalence in a population, the number of contacts of most of the index cases, the resources available for this and other HIV control programs, and the voluntary or mandatory nature of the program (World Health Organization, 1989d). Partner notification is most cost-effective when a partner is unlikely to know she has been exposed to HIV, as in low prevalence populations.

Policymakers must balance these public health benefits against the human rights impact. The burdens depend upon the amount of respect a state gives to the autonomy and privacy of persons with HIV infection and their partners. Partner notification programs which are consistent with human rights principles elicit the informed consent of HIV-infected individuals, do not needlessly disclose their identity, and respect their partners' rights.

Of any program involving the disclosure of HIV-related information, several factors must be rigorously examined. Public officials should consider the groups being tested when the power or the duty to warn is invoked, and the unexpected or untoward consequences. Targeting only a few vulnerable groups for partner notification may discrimi nate and may place individuals at risk of physical harm. This cautions against an exclusive focus on commercial sex workers, for example.

Other groups as well may suffer negative consequences from disclosure. A pregnant woman, for instance, whose partner is notified may blame her for infecting him or their children, even if the woman had been monogamous and was infected by her partner (Hamblin, Reid, 1991). Where health care providers insist on informing women's partners that they have been exposed, privacy, autonomy, and even physical well-being may be compromised. Increasingly, women have reported being abused, beaten, or shot by their partners after the women's HIV status is disclosed. Consequently, some commentators have urged health care providers to weigh carefully the risks of imminent harm to the woman against any possible public health benefits when deciding whether to inform a partner (North, Rothenberg, 1993).

Conclusion

From a human rights perspective, the key factors in programs of casefinding and epidemiologic surveillance are voluntariness, confidentiality, and nondiscrimination. Voluntary testing, reporting, and partner notification can be integral to effective prevention and care programs. Yet, policymakers must be attentive to human rights infringements, not only to ensure dignity but to safeguard the public health.

TRAVEL AND IMMIGRATION RESTRICTIONS

Introduction

Many countries promulgate policies that try to limit the international movement of persons with HIV infection or AIDS. In some cases, formal restrictions are enacted into law or authorized by regulation (Curran, Gostin, et al., 1991; Tomasevski, Gruskin, et al., 1992). In others, no formal policy exists, but practices include requiring "HIV-free certificates" or other travel restrictions (United Nations, 1991; Duckett, Orkin, 1989). This section examines several limitations on freedom of movement by applying the Human Rights Impact Assessment (Chapter 3).

Governments often justify their travel and immigration policies on public health and economic grounds. Specifically, they suggest that restrictions may prevent the spread of HIV to other countries and limit seroprevalence in countries that already harbor the virus. Some also assert the right to protect their citizens from bearing the potential financial burden of persons with chronic illness. On closer inspection, however, such restrictions appear unlikely to achieve their objectives. Furthermore, such measures may actually hinder efforts to control the spread of HIV/AIDS and to mitigate its impact.

The extraordinary volume of international travel, the norm in this century, undoubtedly contributed to the initial spread of HIV (Levine, 1986). At this point in time, though, several reasons suggest that limiting the movement of persons with HIV would not effectively control the virus's spread or the pandemic's growth; HIV infection is already established throughout the world (Porter, Stryker, et al., 1992; Mann, Tarantola, et al., 1992). First restrictive approaches fail to reduce the overall reservoir of infection, nor do they supply needed resources for education and counseling. Second, restrictive policies may erroneously convey that HIV is transmitted through casual contact when, in fact, HIV is spread only through sexual intercourse, exposure to contaminated blood, pregnancy, birth, and breast-feeding. Third, countries cannot safeguard their populations from HIV disease by barricading their borders (Mann, Tarantola, et al., 1992), particularly in countries that already have a substantial number of seropositive individuals. At best, widespread barriers to interstate movement would marginally limit the spread of HIV.

Although world attention has focused on screening international travelers, most restrictions actually target migrant workers, applicants for long-term residence, and returning nationals. Some countries target international students, immigrants, business travelers, asylum seekers, and refugees (Tomasevski, Gruskin, et al., 1992).

The structure of current screening programs for travelers and immigrants casts further doubt on public health justifications. Many policies fail to provide education or counseling necessary to prevent high-risk behavior. The absence of these crucial provisions suggests that the programs neither intend to reduce global HIV transmission, nor will. Moreover, screening or excluding potential immigrants may create a false sense of security among residents; contrary to public health aims, citizens may be less likely to modify behaviors that put them at risk of infection.

Public officials should compare the relative efficacy of restrictions on movement to other programs. Most countries face scarce resources for health protection and promotion, so the opportunity costs of a certain policy matter. Efforts to enforce travel or immigration barriers may consume valuable resources while minimally reducing HIV transmission. Testing is expensive and time-consuming. Since hundreds of millions of people cross international borders annually, testing all or a significant number of them would divert considerable sums away from prevention, education, and treatment programs (World Health Organization, 1987f). Also, mass screening poses serious logistical and technical problems. These include quality control, the potential for false positives, and repeated screening of persons who frequently cross borders.

Policymakers should ensure that their efforts are well targeted. That is, policies should affect only those persons who pose a risk of infection. Restricting freedom of movement solely because a person has HIV infection is inherently overinclusive. By testing all travelers and potential immigrants, and excluding those who are infected, a government bars entry to far more people than necessary to achieve its aim. This policy fails to distinguish between the majority of persons with HIV infection who would act safely and the minority who may not and might pose a risk of transmitting the virus.

The International Health Regulations (1985) prohibit national laws, regulations, or practices that require HIV-antibody testing of persons seeking to enter or leave a country or that condition entry upon "HIV-free certificates." Pursuant to the Regulations, the only document that may be required for international travel is a valid certificate of vaccination against yellow fever (World Health Organization, 1992d; see also Chapter 1: Freedom of Movement). In practice, governments have disregarded the International Health Regulations without any formal international consequences. But publicity and domestic pressure over time may act as a check on some government violations of international law (see also Chapter 1). American refusal to allow Haitians with HIV infection to enter the country (despite valid claims for political asylum) exemplifies the exclusionary policies that some governments have adopted. An initial domestic court order enabled some Haitians to enter the United States, but a higher court later reversed the decision (Greenhouse, 1993). The broader ban prohibiting persons with HIV infection from entering the country under most circumstances (as immigrants or long-term residents) remains in place (Krauss, 1993).

On the other hand, countries have no general obligation to allow entry by nonnationals (with certain exceptions for asylum seekers and refugees) (see Chapter 1: Freedom of Movement, and references to specific policies below). International documents explicitly guarantee only the right to freedom of movement *within one's own country* and the right to *leave one's country and subsequently return* (UDHR, Art. 13; ICCPR, Art. 12). However, denying entry to individuals based solely on HIV infection fundamentally infringes on human rights. First, preventing international movement by persons with HIV infection substantially affects a broad scope of human endeavors, including family unity; business, cultural, and scientific exchange; and access to specialized health care. Second, restrictions may also interfere with international cooperation among scientists, activists, and persons with HIV/AIDS. For example, in 1990, United States officials attempted to bar some San Francisco AIDS Conference participants from entering the country. When the United States federal government announced its intention to continue to bar foreigners with HIV infection from entering the country, the 1992 AIDS Conference organizers relocated the Conference from Boston to Amsterdam. Third, one country's restriction may lead other countries to retaliate with their own limitations. Lastly, testing and excluding persons based on HIV infection alone is a form of "status" discrimination. Unless justified by a compelling reason and based upon reasonable and objective criteria, such policies offend the nondiscrimination principles articulated in the International Bill of Human Rights and countless other international documents (United Nations, 1995a,b; Rights and Humanity Declaration, 1992). Behavior, not serologic status, is the relevant criterion in the HIV/AIDS context, because the disease is not casually transmitted.

Screening and excluding foreigners may also violate individuals' right to privacy. Policies that share HIV test results among government agencies, private parties, or states offend privacy rights. Only a compelling justification could sustain such approaches (see also Chapter 1: Privacy, and this chapter, Epidemiological Surveillance and Disease Control).

In addition to public health rationales, governments may restrict interstate movement on economic grounds, explicitly or implicitly. States may seek to avoid caring for a non-national with a serious illness. However, testing policies that discriminate against persons with disabilities may violate international covenants (Dickens, Howe, et al., 1992). Moreover, testing solely to exclude persons from services departs from public health traditions (Gostin, Cleary, et al., 1990). If governments were genuinely concerned with cost, they would bar all persons with chronic diseases that require expensive treatments (such as heart or kidney disease, or cancer). Many persons seeking to immigrate to a country have family or other ties there. To prevent such a person from joining a spouse, parents, or children precisely because of ill health is troubling.

Impacts of Travel and Immigration Restrictions

Restricting freedom of movement violates the International Health Regulations (1985) and significantly burdens basic human rights. If states routinely applied testing and exclusion policies to all persons who sought to cross international borders, the scope of human rights violations would be enormous. Individuals with HIV infection would endure life-long burdens on human rights, including the rights to family unity, work, education, and free exchange of information, particularly scientific and medical knowledge and advances. Moreover, such burdens would extend to future generations; children would suffer from broken families, from their parent's inability to obtain work or necessary treatment, and from stigmatization as a result of exclusion. By contrast, the public health benefits of restricting movement of persons with HIV infection are minimal—both from a global and state perspective. Given the few benefits and multiple burdens of this approach, policymakers should consider alternatives.

To highlight particular impacts on human rights and public health, we now examine how entry barriers affect different groups.

Travelers

Most of the hundreds of millions of persons who cross international borders every day are short-term travelers and others who do not require visas. Comprehensive programs to screen all short-term travelers pose significant logistical difficulties and opportunity costs. Therefore, efforts to screen travelers are likely to be selective and thus to discriminate by race, national or geographic origin, perceived sexual orientation, or occupation. Such testing exacerbates existing misconceptions and prejudices about HIV. In its Statement on Screening of International Travellers for Infection with Human Immunodeficiency Virus (1988g), the World Health Organization concluded that screening is ineffective, impractical, and wasteful.

Immigrants and long-term residents

States may target immigrants, visa applicants, and long-term-residency permit-seekers for testing. Alternatively, they may require certificates demonstrating the absence of infection, foreseeably leading to a market in counterfeit "HIV-free certificates." Moreover, persons at risk of infection may attempt to enter a country illegally, with attendant risks to their health, liberty, security of person, and, perhaps, life. If already illegally present, persons at risk may avoid contact with health and social services because of fear that their infection status might be detected and reported to government authorities.

Migrant workers and foreign students

Border personnel often screen migrant workers and foreign students for HIV regardless of official authorization (Tomasevski, Gruskin, et al., 1992). The majority of persons infected with HIV fall within an economically productive age group (World Health Organization, 1988f, 1991) (e.g., agricultural or industrial or service-sector workers or students pursuing secondary or higher education abroad). For most, HIV infection does not impair their ability to work or study productively.

Estimates suggest that nearly ninety percent of the projected HIV infections this decade will occur in developing countries (World Health Organization, 1992). Since vast numbers of persons cross international borders every year to work or study, the economic and social impact of such restrictions could be quite broad.

Barriers to entry would deprive individuals of the benefits of income or knowledge acquired abroad. This harms the economy and infrastructure of workers' and students' home countries, which might otherwise benefit from their earnings and technical or professional training. The burden would be especially heavy for developing countries that depend on migrant workers to introduce foreign currency, and on foreign universities to train many of their skilled professionals.

Returning nationals

Testing returning nationals is misguided for several reasons. First, authorities cannot distinguish between people who were infected prior to travel and those who became infected abroad. Second, such testing raises basic issues of fairness. Excluding, isolating, or otherwise punishing persons regardless of where they were infected is manifestly unfair. Third, such an approach might chill travel for business, medical, scientific, or other reasons. Moreover, a state that denies reentry to infected nationals is violating fundamental human rights (UDHR, Art. 13; ICCPR, Art. 12).

Refugees and asylum seekers

Both persons seeking asylum (those already within a country) and those claiming refugee status (those abroad who wish to enter a country) must present a well-founded fear of persecution in their home countries. The determination of refugee status and the decision to grant asylum contain an element of discretion which should be limited to the facts surrounding an individual's safety in his home country. In practice, political, ideological, and economic considerations influence these determinations.

International documents protect asylum seekers and refugees. Testing and excluding asylum-seekers on the basis of HIV infection violates the Universal Declaration of Human Rights, which guarantees to everyone the right to seek and enjoy in other countries asylum from persecution (Art. 14). Neither the 1951 Convention nor the 1967 Protocol on the Status of Refugees addressed the issue of refugees who are chronically ill or disabled. Testing for HIV infection that leads to denial of refugee status, to refusal of entry by third countries, to forcible return, or to barred entry to the country of origin is morally and legally suspect. These discriminatory policies conflict with the principles that guide international efforts to resettle refugees—namely, "non-refoulement [no driving back (of refugees)] and durable solutions premised upon international co-operation and solidarity." Consequently, the United Nations High Commissioner for Refugees (UNHCR) has opposed mass testing of refugees and has urged that refugees are given access to the same levels of voluntary testing, counseling, and care that are available to nationals (UNHCR, 1988).

Testing of both asylum-seekers and refugees targets particularly vulnerable groups—those fleeing persecution. Additionally, some of those denied asylum or refuge may be placed in grave danger; forcing them to return to their country of origin may threaten their right liberty and even their lives (see Chapter 1: The Right to Life).

Long-term detention of persons with HIV infection

A few countries have established mass screening programs for their own populations. Cuba, for instance, has tested a substantial portion of its population and has confined all those infected with HIV to sanitaria (Bayer, Healton, 1989). Although most Cubans with HIV are now allowed to leave the sanitaria to visit friends and family, the restriction on liberty remains substantial and life-long. Other governments authorize the indefinite isolation or hospitalization of persons with HIV infection for "compulsory treatment" (United Nations, 1991). In addition to infringing on the right to liberty, these policies burden HIV-infected persons' right to move freely within their own country, contrary to international law (UDHR, Art. 13; ICCPR, Art. 12).

Less Restrictive Policies

Given the marginal public health benefit, the probable public health harms, and the significant human rights burdens of limiting the movement of persons with HIV infection, public officials should consider less restrictive alternatives. Other policies—such as education, counseling, and voluntary testing—are more appropriate for people who cross international borders. Educating people about the risks of HIV infection encourages them to protect themselves (and others) from possible transmission during sexual intercourse or drug use. Voluntary testing based on informed consent respects individual dignity and autonomy; simultaneously, it allows persons who wish to know their HIV status to do so without fear of "punishment" via denied entry. Those who seek to immigrate to, or who already reside in, another country would not have to remain "underground" if they suspected they might be infected. People who feared persecution in their own country would not have to choose between remaining in danger or seeking asylum in a country where they might be confined indefinitely if found to be infected.

Each of these alternatives potentially prevents new infections, uses resources wisely, and encourages cooperation between government authorities and persons who might have HIV infection.

THE HEALTH CARE SYSTEM

Introduction

Approximately five percent of HIV infections worldwide are caused by contaminated blood or blood products (Beal, Britten, et al., 1992). Health care professionals' exposure to HIV through injury with contaminated instruments or lack of effective barrier precautions (masks, gloves) probably represents a much smaller proportion. Transmissions of HIV through the blood supply or within the medical workplace are perhaps the most preventable, because the population at risk is clearly identifiable, and relatively low-cost, effective precautionary measures are available. Actual prevention, however, depends upon states' efforts to educate individuals at risk; maintain an adequate, safe supply of blood and donated organs; and provide and promote health care workers' use of sterile equipment and protective clothing. Individuals alone lack the resources and technical expertise to implement and enforce prevention measures. Particularly in emergency situations, a transfusion recipient often has no alternative but to accept whatever blood supplies are available. Health care workers in many settings must choose between providing life-saving care without adequately protecting themselves or having sterile supplies for the patients, or not providing the care.

Several human rights principles impose on states an affirmative duty to protect blood recipients. Individuals have a right to share in the benefits of science and technology, including proven protective measures (screened blood, gloves, masks). Failure to ensure a safe blood supply and access to sterile medical equipment and protective measures burdens the rights to health and life.

Patients who know they may require blood transfusions during a medical procedure may plan in advance to store and use their own blood ("autologous" transfusions). However, this is an exceptional case, and patients need objective and timely information in order to exercise this option. The inherent dignity and worth of every individual entitles him to make health care decisions informed by the potential benefits and risks.

Blood Supply

Patients are at serious risk of illness or death when blood supplies for medically necessary transfusions are inadequate or unsafe. Patients may die from a loss of blood that reserves cannot replenish, from postponement of necessary surgery, or from a fatal infection from a tainted transfusion. Serious (but not always fatal) diseases such as hepatitis, syphilis, and malaria may also be transmitted. Current estimates indicate that annually eighty million units of blood are collected and transfused worldwide; all countries should be concerned about the potential for substantial harm (Britten, 1988). The international market in blood, blood products, and, to a lesser extent, other tissues efficiently spreads HIV and other blood-borne pathogens through untested or untreated products. Like pharmaceuticals, these "goods" are imported and exported. A health care system with inadequate safety procedures thus poses a risk to its own citizens as well as to others who import the product. Early in the AIDS epidemic, for example, HIV was transmitted to persons with hemophilia through contaminated imported blood products (Riding, 1994; Hunter, 1993).

The World Health Organization has recommended that all countries establish and maintain integrated transfusion services, promote the use of safe blood and sterile equipment, and restrict injections and skin-piercing procedures to medically necessary situations (World Health Organization, 1988h, 1989i, 1987h). In addition, in 1988, the Global Blood Safety Initiative was launched by the League of Red Cross and Red Crescent Societies (LRCRCS), the United Nations Development Programme (UNDP), the International Society of Blood Transfusion (ISBT), and the World Federation Hemophilia (WFH). This project aims to secure in all countries accessible, appropriate, adequate, and safe blood supplies. At least fifty countries have enacted laws or regulations that require blood donor screening or testing for HIV and other infectious agents (Curran, Gostin, et al., 1991). Unfortunately, in practice many developing countries lack the resources, equipment, and trained personnel to screen every donated unit for HIV, hepatitis B, or a host of other agents (World Health Organization, 1987i; N'tita, Mulanga, et al., 1991).

Governments should consider four methods to prevent transfusion or transplant-related HIV infection. These include donor selection, laboratory testing, appropriate use of blood, and viral inactivation. These approaches are interdependent; a government cannot ignore one without reducing the efficacy of the others (Beal, Britten, et al., 1992). Below, we examine each intervention, evaluate its efficacy, and assess its potential impact on human rights.[1]

---

1. For more information about the program, consult the national or international organizations that are cooperating with the Global Blood Safety Initiative.

Donor selection

Donor screening procedures seek to minimize the proportion of blood donors with HIV infection. No system of donor selection is 100 percent effective. A carefully designed process, however, can significantly safeguard the blood supply through education and counseling, screening, and recruitment of voluntary donors (Schutz, Savarit, et al., 1993). Prospective donors must be informed about possible risk factors for HIV infection and defer donation if they are at risk. Policies should ensure confidentiality of donation and deferral to all prospective donors.

Many countries do not have a sufficient pool of voluntary donors to meet their current demands for blood. Industrialized and developing countries often differ greatly with respect to their donors. In industrialized nations, unpaid volunteers supply most of the blood; in developing states, most blood donations come from family, friends, or paid donors (Beal, Britten, et al., 1992). Historically, many countries have relied upon paid donors for blood, blood products, or gametes. Monetary payments have even been linked to organ donation. Evidence suggests that remunerated donors have higher rates of infectious disease than do voluntary donors. For instance, rates of hepatitis B infection are reportedly three times higher among paid donors than among unpaid (United States, 1975); hepatitis C infection is twenty-eight times higher in paid donors than unpaid (United States, 1991); and HIV infection seventy times higher in paid donors than unpaid (Mexico, 1989) (Beal, Britten, et al., 1992). Some voluntary donors, particularly those recruited among family or friends, have a measurably higher rate of HIV infection than mass volunteer donors.

Studies have led countries to shift recruitment and retention efforts to voluntary donors and to reduce reliance on paid donors (Beal, Britten, et al., 1992). Some countries are exploring strategies for recruiting voluntary blood donors. The human rights implications of this change are clear: States must educate the public on the need for donations. To attract and retain blood donors, States must ensure their safety by using sterile equipment and by meticulously adhering to infection-control procedures. Even where safe blood donation procedures are well established, fears and misconceptions may reduce voluntary donations. In addition, states should consider the needs of persons who formerly depended upon paid donations for income. States might offer job-training for former paid donors, provide social security for those who became infected while donating, and initiate other measures that reduce these persons' economic reliance on blood donation.

Donor selection programs may involve human rights by the way in which they define "risk factors" or conditions for self-deferral. Population-based deferral criteria, such as ethnicity or race, are a particular concern. Such classifications constitute status discrimination, which all the major human rights declarations and covenants prohibit (see Chapter 1: Nondiscrimination). Proper deferral criteria should be solidly grounded in scientific and behavioral studies.

In societies that have a high seroprevalence among all sexually active adults, it may not be possible to identify adequate criteria for self-deferral while ensuring a sufficient supply of voluntary donors. Given the critical importance of a safe blood supply and the strain caused by HIV/AIDS on many societies' resources, international assistance may be required. Under the UDHR and ICESCR, states pledge to share technology, particularly when necessary to realize economic, social, and cultural rights in countries with few resources. The ethical principle of distributive justice requires that benefits and burdens be shared fairly (Beauchamp, Childress, 1994). When poorer populations face serious risks from contaminated blood supplies, countries that are better able to promote such approaches are ethically obligated to provide some level of assistance.

Laboratory testing

Researchers first developed the HIV-antibody test for use in blood banks. Today, its use on donated blood is virtually universally accepted due to the test's relative accuracy, the effectiveness and ease of using the results, and the potential for well-designed programs that burden human rights minimally, if at all.

States should test all blood, tissues, and organs for HIV antibodies, hepatitis B, and other infectious agents. When properly performed, these tests are quite accurate (Brandt, Cleary, et al., 1990). Several sources of possible error exist in testing blood for HIV. First, since the test detects antibodies rather than virus, potential donors who were recently infected may test negative because they have not yet developed antibodies to HIV. The second source of error is false-negative tests. As with any laboratory test, some blood samples that contain antibodies will show negative results. In the United States, the risk of HIV transmission from a unit of blood that has falsely tested negative is currently estimated to be one in 450,000–600,000 (Lackritz, Satten, et al., 1995), lower than earlier estimates of one in 68,000 (Kleinman, Secord, 1988; Ward, Holmberg, et al., 1988). In contrast, where a particularly high incidence (occurrence of new infections) exists among blood donors, the risk can be far greater. One study in West Africa estimated that even after screening, the risk of a unit of blood being HIV-infected was 5.4 per 1,000 units (Savarit, DeCock, et al., 1992). The test best safeguards the blood supply where donor selection policies minimize the number of donors likely to be infected. Finally, the identification of distinct HIV-1 subtypes has caused concern that tests developed for antibodies to one subtype may not detect blood contaminated with other subtypes. In 1996, the Centers for Disease Control and Prevention reported that blood from an HIV-infected patient with a subtype rare in the United States did not test positive for antibodies using several of the commercially available tests relied upon by U.S. blood banks (Centers for Disease Control and Prevention, 1996).

Test results should unequivocally lead to effective state action to reduce the risk of transmission. Health officials should ensure that all blood, tissues, organs, or other products that test positive are discarded, even where a positive test cannot be confirmed.

A carefully designed testing program for donated blood and tissues raises minimal human rights concerns. Prospective donors should know before they donate their blood that it will be tested for HIV antibodies and other infectious agents. This preserves informed consent principles, maintains conditional donation, and rests upon implied consent to testing. Blood which initially tests positive for HIV antibodies should undergo additional tests to confirm the results. Donors should receive positive test results in a timely manner, as well as education, counseling, and access to appropriate social services.

Human rights concerns may arise over how states handle the intimate personal data collected by the blood bank. HIV test results and information on drug use and sexual behavior deserve the highest degree of privacy protection. Breaches of confidentiality may inflict substantial personal harm if the information is shared with other government agencies or private parties (see Chapter 1: Privacy; and this chapter, Epidemiological Surveillance and Disease Control).

Similar public health issues arise in the donation of tissues, organs, and gametes. The public must be apprised of the demand for donated tissue. In most countries that possess the technical expertise to support organ transplantation, demand for donated organs and tissues far outstrips supply. States should screen potential donors for known risk factors, and, where feasible, should perform HIV-antibody tests prior to using the tissues, organs, or gametes.

Appropriate usage

The inappropriate use of blood and blood products remains a serious problem worldwide. The WHO estimates that twenty to twenty-five percent of red blood cell transfusions and up to ninety percent of the albumin used in industrialized countries may be unnecessary (World Health Organization, 1987i). In Africa, strict criteria governing the proper use of blood has reduced transfusions by sixty percent in some institutions. Eliminating, or at least lowering, the incidence of blood misuse would reduce transfusion-related disease (DeCock, Ekpini, et al., 1994). Moreover, it would conserve scarce resources, thereby increasing the safety and quantity of blood available for life-saving transfusions. Thus, the state has an affirmative duty to educate health care workers about the appropriate uses of blood and to discourage improper uses.

Viral inactivation

Preparation processes by heat treatment of certain blood products (e.g., plasma, Factors VIII and IX, immune serum globulin, and others treatment) can inactivate viruses. Failure to implement such steps have tragically affected persons with hemophilia, many of whom were infected with HIV through contaminated blood factors. The decision by

French government officials knowingly to distribute—rather than to destroy—contaminated blood factors led to a court judgment, the removal or resignation of government ministers, and continuing public controversy over the preventable infection of many persons with hemophilia (Riding, 1994; Hunter, 1993). The officials' failure caused not only severe physical harm but violated the trust of those who depended on the state for information about the safety of the blood supply and medications.

Patient Testing and Screening

In many countries, patients in the health care system have been the first populations to undergo screening for HIV (Tomasevski, Gruskin, et al., 1992). Programs have targeted patients in hospitals and those attending prenatal, primary care, sexually transmitted infection (STI), and other clinics. (For a more detailed discussion of issues surrounding testing, see this chapter, Epidemiological Surveillance and Disease Control.)

Evaluating such testing and screening programs from a human rights perspective requires assessing (1) the coercive or voluntary nature of the program, (2) the public health objectives of screening and whether they will be achieved, and (3) the privacy safeguards for patients.

Level of coercion in testing

Public officials may conduct testing or screening programs with various levels of coercion. Voluntary testing with a person's informed consent fully respects autonomy and generally does not burden human rights. Compulsory testing or screening without consent is based on the state's power to override personal autonomy; it therefore requires the most compelling justification. Routine screening programs, while not inherently coercive, may not adequately allow the patient to make a truly informed choice. Systematically screening all hospital patients without fully informing them and seeking their consent *before* testing does not constitute voluntary HIV testing. Health care facilities' screening of patients' blood after removing all identifying information—and use of the results solely for research or epidemiological purposes—has been accepted and endorsed by many public health organizations and ethicists. (For more on blinded or anonymous screening, see this chapter, Epidemiological Surveillance and Disease Control.)

Objectives of testing: clinical, public health, occupational safety

Testing or screening patients for HIV infection requires evaluating the objectives and determining whether they can be achieved. Common justifications for screening or testing patients include clinical benefits for individuals, improved public health for the community, and occupational safety for health care professionals.

Many health care professionals believe that the primary purpose of testing is to benefit patients. In many areas, particularly more developed countries, professionals can offer antiviral medications such as zidovudine (AZT), an expanding array of antiretroviral medications, and prophylactic treatments for opportunistic infections such as pneumocystis carinii pneumonia. In developing countries or those experiencing economic turmoil, doctors or healers may advise improved nutrition or offer traditional medicines.

The desire to help persons with HIV infection is commendable. Nevertheless, under most international ethical codes, patients have the right to decide for themselves whether they want even the most beneficial treatments (CIOMS, 1991, 1993). Health care providers and public health authorities cannot justifiably override the express wishes of competent, adult patients exclusively on the basis of their perception of the best interests of the patient. Respect for human beings means allowing them to decide for themselves where their interests lie. Many societies allow exceptions to this principle for children and noncompetent adults.

In parts of Africa and other communal societies in the South and East, persons who are young or very sick may be tested or treated for their own benefit regardless of their wishes (Ankrah, Gostin, 1994). Respect for a society's cultural values is critical. Often, however, both respect for individual autonomy and communitarian values can be accommodated. In such cases, the professional or healer and the patient may consult family members, elders, and leaders on a confidential basis. Patients then should make their own decisions guided by persons they trust.

Testing patients with their informed consent is desirable not only from a human rights perspective but also from a public health perspective. The process of discussing the purpose and implications of HIV testing offers a prime opportunity to assess risk, to counsel, and to educate about behavior modification. Patients become partners in a therapeutic process only when health care providers consult them and honor their wishes.

In addition to the potential clinical benefits of screening patients for HIV, officials often justify such policies on public health grounds. Some argue that screening for HIV infection imparts crucial information to patients, which in turn effects behavioral change and slows HIV transmission. Voluntary testing of persons who engage in high-risk behavior, accompanied by pre- and post-test counseling and education, can be an effective prevention strategy (Higgins, Galavotti, et al., 1991). However, testing a person without consent or counseling is unlikely to protect the public health. Insufficient data exist regarding how knowledge of HIV test results alone affect behavior. Consent, counseling, and education constitute fundamental parts of a sound prevention strategy. Indeed, compulsory measures may be counterproductive to public health goals: Fear may drive persons at greatest risk of infection away from the health care system.

Some health professionals seek to test patients for HIV primarily to protect the workers themselves, rather than the patients or the community (see Chapter 1: Privacy). Their fears are understandable, especially if they work in high-seroprevalence areas. It is unclear, however, whether the knowledge gained by involuntary testing of patients would help providers protect themselves. The actual risk of HIV infection after percutaneous exposure to HIV-infected blood is relatively low, approximately 0.03 percent (Centers for Disease Control and Prevention, 1994a). These numbers do not reflect a health care provider's cumulative or lifetime risk of repeated exposures. Studies in some countries show significant rates of needlestick injuries, particularly during invasive procedures and trauma care. Several hundred cases of occupationally contracted HIV infection among health care workers have been reported worldwide. Despite these legitimate concerns, the WHO (1987j) has concluded that health care workers are at very low risk of occupationally acquired infection. Adherence to strict infection control procedures ("universal precautions") can further lower the risk.

The central question is whether routine or compulsory testing of patients is an effective strategy to reduce the health care workers' risk of occupational exposure. No evidence to date demonstrates that if health care workers were informed of their patients' serostatus, that they could take any precautions that would reduce their risk. Since HIV testing does not detect all patients with HIV infection, health care workers might be at a heightened risk if they rely on test results to identify patients who pose a risk of infection and they fail to maintain rigorous infection-control measures with all patients. In most of the reported cases of HIV transmission to health care workers, the professionals already knew the patient's HIV status. Most of the exposures occurred after accidental needlestick injuries or mucous membrane exposures to large quantities of contaminated blood. Awareness of the risk of infection did not appear to prevent transmission in these cases.

In June 1996, the U.S. Public Health Service published provisional recommendations for chemoprophylaxis of health care or other workers after occupational exposure to HIV (Centers for Disease Control and Prevention, 1996a). The recommendations are based on evidence that taking zidovudine (ZDV) after percutaneous or mucous membrane exposure to HIV-infected blood may reduce the likelihood of infection (Centers for Disease Control and Prevention, 1995g). These recommendations suggest that exposed workers begin treatment with ZDV, another antiretroviral drug such as 3TC, and a protease inhibitor, preferably indinavir (IDV), within one to two hours of exposure and continuing for four weeks postexposure. The full regimen is recommended for percutaneous exposures (especially those involving visible blood or deep injury to the worker). The same or a similar regimen should be offered, along with full counseling about the potential risks and benefits, to workers with lower risk exposures. The Public Health Service provisional recommendations do not mention compulsory testing of source patients. They advise exposed workers only that if the patient's HIV status is unknown, the worker should make decisions about prophylaxis on a case-by-case basis based on exposure risk and likelihood of HIV infection in the source. If additional information becomes available (e.g., source patient consents to testing) the worker and his or her health care provider can modify decisions about postexposure prophylaxis (Centers for Disease Control and Prevention, 1996a). Pursuant to these recommendations, testing of all patients is neither contemplated nor necessary. Assuming that workers can begin prophylaxis based on other information allows health care workers to seek consent from the source patient for testing and confirmation of HIV status, or, where the source patient is unidentifiable or refuses testing, to continue prophylactic treatment without conclusive evidence. Such a policy takes aggressive steps both to ensure the health of potentially exposed workers and to protect the autonomy, privacy, and security of patients.

When considering routine or compulsory testing or screening of patients, policymakers should ask what the objectives are and whether screening achieves them most effectively. The principal benefits of screening are usually the accompanying counseling, education, treatment, and care. These gains depend on a therapeutic partnership that only the patient's consent and active participation can secure.

Privacy safeguards afforded to patients

Testing or screening programs involving patients must protect the confidentiality of test results. A person's HIV status is highly personal information. When a patient discusses his or her intimate behavior with a health care worker and is tested for HIV infection, an implicit or explicit promise exists to keep that information confidential. Disclosure without the patient's consent may cause serious economic harm, such as loss of employment or employability, insurance or insurability, or housing. Disclosure may also result in social and psychological harms including stigmatization, embarrassment, social isolation, and loss of self-esteem. Family members, neighbors, and fellow workers may withdraw social support. Therefore, in assessing the human rights aspects of testing and screening programs, policymakers should give close attention to safeguarding the privacy of patients (see Chapter 2: Confidentiality and Privacy).

Access to Health Care and Discrimination

Persons with HIV or AIDS often experience difficulty in obtaining affordable health care. Potential barriers to services include economic class, gender, race, culture, and language differences as well as discrimination on the basis of HIV infection.

Public officials worldwide must facilitate access to health care for persons with HIV infection. Wherever possible, primary care practitioners, rather than specialists in university or teaching hospitals, should treat persons with HIV disease. Programs should provide basic services through primary care providers and routine follow-up located near patients' homes. This expands the number of people with access to care and promotes treatment in cost-effective settings, such as the home rather than the hospital. Programs should ensure care to people in urban areas, prisons, homeless shelters, STI and drug clinics, and in rural or tribal areas that lack adequate health care facilities. The need for accessible care is particularly great among underserved populations such as the poor, ethnic minorities, and women.

Denying patients care because of their HIV status can pose serious health risks to individuals. Even when such discrimination causes little or no physical harm, it demonstrates a lack of respect and empathy that violates most standards of professional conduct and basic tenets of human rights. When based on the prospective patient's HIV status alone, such differential treatment constitutes discrimination based on status. Unless reasonable or objective criteria *and* a compelling need justify the discrimination, the Universal Declaration of Human Rights and all related Covenants prohibit it. Discrimination based on status burdens human rights both when a health care provider refuses to accept a new patient solely because he has HIV, and when the provider terminates an existing relationship because a patient contracts HIV. Although both acts are discriminatory, moral and professional standards may particularly condemn the latter (e.g., abandoning a patient after establishing an ongoing relationship) (see Chapter 1: Nondiscrimination).

Some health care providers decline to accept patients with HIV infection because they claim to have insufficient expertise to treat HIV-related illnesses. Certainly, some complications of HIV disease require specialized knowledge. Referral to a specialist in these situations is a permissible, and expected, part of medical practice. However, states should not allow exercises of clinical judgment to mask invidious discrimination. All providers should be held responsible for providing the level of expertise prevailing in the community. Therefore, as the seroprevalence increases, health care workers need to develop and maintain minimum standards of care for persons with HIV infection. A health care provider who chooses not to attain this minimum level is discriminating and failing a professional obligation. To determine whether care should have been provided, officials should ask: (1) Would the provider have treated the patient, absent HIV infection? and (2) Is the complexity of the case commensurate with the particular community's expectation of its practitioners?

Health care workers may refuse to provide certain kinds of care because they perceive an occupational risk. The occupational risk of infection to a health care worker from an infected patient is very low, but nonetheless real. Some providers believe that they must provide treatment if necessary to save or prolong a life notwithstanding the risk of infection; however, they reserve the right to decline providing "elective" or cosmetic treatment. Professional practice has not clearly defined "elective" and "cosmetic" procedures, and the definitions imposed by individual providers may be irrelevant to the patient's actual needs and quality of life. For example, the concept of "elective" treatment can be meaningless if the services are necessary to alleviate pain or suffering or to restore function (e.g., to correct a disfigurement that may vastly improve a person's quality of life).

Patients with HIV disease deserve the same quality of care as all other patients. The fundamental question is whether patient X should receive different treatment than patient Y, not because of clinical differences, but because of a perceived occupational risk to the provider. States should tolerate differential treatment only where a procedure poses a substantial risk of infection to the provider and precautionary measures afford insufficient protection. Since the risk of HIV infection to health care providers, including those performing invasive procedures, is low and can be further reduced through infection control procedures (World Health Organization, 1987j), health care workers are ethically obligated to provide treatment within their sphere of experience and expertise.

HIV-Infected Health Care Workers: Testing and Discrimination

Testing providers

The well-publicized case of an American health care worker (a Florida dentist) who appears to have transmitted HIV to six of his patients (Centers for Disease Control and Prevention, 1993) has raised public fears. In some countries, this fear incited calls to screen all health care workers.

The actual risk of a provider infecting a patient is quite low. An investigation of almost 20,000 patients who received treatment from fifty-seven HIV-infected health care workers found no other case of such transmission (Centers for Disease Control and Prevention, 1993).

Health care workers are obligated to provide professional care and not unreasonably to endanger patients who depend upon them. Therefore, providers who might be infected should seek testing voluntarily, and, if infected, should refrain from activities that pose a substantial risk of transmission.

Public health authorities do not recommend compulsory testing of health care workers (Centers for Disease Control and Prevention, 1991a; World Health Organization, 1991b). The extremely small risk of transmission does not justify the substantial diversion of resources that routine or compulsory testing would require. To be effective, providers would have to repeatedly undergo testing, and authorities would have to keep detailed, updated records of HIV status. The potential infringements on individual autonomy, privacy, and confidentiality, and the potential for false positives, exist as in programs for the widespread testing of patients.

Discrimination

Whether testing is voluntary, routine, or compulsory, a question remains regarding appropriate limitations (if any) on the practice of HIV-infected health care workers. A strong argument exists to permit HIV-infected health care workers to continue their normal practice, provided they are able to do so and to follow rigorous infection control procedures. In 1991, the U.S. Centers for Disease Control issued recommendations to prevent transmission of HIV and hepatitis B (HBV) from health care workers to patients. These recommendations emphasized: (1) All health care workers should observe universal precautions. (2) Health care workers infected with HIV who do not perform invasive procedures or do not perform exposure-prone invasive procedures (likely to include the exchange of blood if the health care worker is injured) should not have their practices restricted. (3) Professional organizations and institutions should define "exposure-prone" procedures within their own settings. (4) Health care workers who perform exposure-prone procedures should know their HIV and HBV status. (5) Health care workers who are infected should not perform exposure-prone procedures unless they have sought counsel from an expert review panel and been advised under what conditions they may do so. (6) Those conditions should include notifying prospective patients prior to the procedure (Centers for Disease Control and Prevention, 1991a).

Barring HIV-infected health care professionals from practice substantially burdens their rights. They may lose their livelihood when in fact they pose little or no threat to patients. They may also suffer emotional and psychological harm from disclosure of their HIV status to patients and colleagues. Additionally, such exclusion may constitute a significant waste of resources in areas that already have a shortage of care-giving personnel. Such restrictions must be justified by an individualized determination that the person poses a significant risk to his or her patients.

In many ways, HIV disease has transformed the health care system. Patients and health care workers each claim a right to know the HIV status of the other. Calls for screening and exclusion undermine the trust and sense of caring required between health care workers and patients. To enhance both public health and human rights, health care workers and the public should treat HIV disease more like other illnesses where affected persons receive nurturing and care rather than stigmatization.

PERSONAL CONTROL MEASURES

Introduction

In many countries, the response to the HIV/AIDS epidemic has been strikingly similar. Typically, the first impulse is to deny that HIV/AIDS poses a risk in that country. Once the first signs of the epidemic are observed and the population realizes the risk of infection, the reaction is often panic, accompanied by pressure on the government to protect the citizenry (Commonwealth Secretariat, 1990). In addition to early calls for mass screening, authorities have invoked coercive powers. Proposals have included isolation or confinement of persons with HIV infection, monitoring or surveillance, criminalization of HIV transmission, and legal sanctions against persons assumed to be HIV "carriers" (e.g., drug users, homosexuals, and commercial sex workers). This section examines each of these policies from both the human rights and the public health perspective with reference to the Human Rights Impact Assessment (Chapter 3).

Isolation, Quarantine, and Compulsory Treatment

At least seventeen countries have adopted legal measures to isolate, quarantine, or confine people with HIV infection or AIDS. Some countries justify such laws or policies as "compulsory treatment" or as medically necessary (Tomasevski, Gruskin, et al., 1992). Many other jurisdictions apply general communicable disease statutes to test, examine, or confine persons with HIV infection without their consent. Drafted in earlier eras of infectious disease control, many of these public health statutes and regulations are inconsistent with both modern disease control measures and human/ civil rights (Gostin, 1986, 1993). Their focus on physically separating infected and noninfected individuals is inappropriate for HIV/AIDS, since the virus is not casually transmitted and generally depends on voluntary behavior for both transmission and prevention. Moreover, these older statutes often give authorities broad discretion to confine individuals, but they neither provide a graduated series of powers nor require the use of the least restrictive alternative. The World Health Assembly (1992, 1989, 1988, 1987) and the WHO (1987a) maintain that no public health rationale justifies isolation, quarantine, or other discriminatory measures based solely on HIV infection (see also United Nations, 1995a, 1994a).

Coercive measures for HIV control under older communicable disease statutes or newer HIV-specific statutes are generally ineffective and seriously burden human rights. Restrictions that apply to all persons with HIV infection are broader than necessary to achieve the public health purpose of containing the infection; they affect, in addition to the few persons who pose a risk of infection, many persons who do not. More focused interventions apply only to HIV-infected persons who engage in defined behaviors such as unprotected sex or sharing of contaminated injection equipment. But even these are often counterproductive for public health. Imposing coercive measures, especially those that involve a significant loss of liberty, discourages trust and cooperation between public health authorities and the community. Moreover, it also does not promote the voluntary behavior change that is necessary to control the spread of HIV. Indeed, fear of coercion may deter people at risk from seeking testing or treatment. Fear of coercive measures can drive people likely to be infected with HIV away from the health care system. Finally, such approaches often reflect an underlying public attitude—that persons with HIV infection pose a danger to society. This view stigmatizes people living with HIV/ AIDS and exacerbates the fears and discrimination directed against them.

International human rights guarantee to protect the liberty and security of the individual from arbitrary arrest or detention (UDHR, Art. 9; ICCPR, Art. 9). These doctrines require that lawfully detained individuals receive humane treatment and not be handled in a cruel, inhuman, or degrading manner (UDHR, Art. 5; ICCPR, Art. 7, 10). State measures to isolate, quarantine, or compulsorily treat persons with HIV infection substantially burden these basic human rights. Compulsory state measures that restrict individual liberty may also infringe on freedom of association (by all forms of detention) and on privacy and security of person (by compulsory medical examinations or "treatment"). Depending on the conditions of confinement, a government's use of coercive powers may violate the right to humane treatment (see Chapter 1: Freedom from Arbitrary Arrest, Detention, or Exile; Right to Security; Privacy; Freedom from Inhumane and Degrading Treatment).

Under specific circumstances, protection of the public health may justify burdening an individual's right to liberty or other fundamental rights (UDHR, Art. 2a; ICCPR, Art. 4, 9, 18, 19, 21). The Siracusa Principles (1984) seek to clarify the criteria for derogation of human rights on public health grounds: the law provides for it, a compelling public health need exists, and the derogation is the least restrictive alternative that accomplishes the public health goal. Additionally, jurisprudence in the mental health area contains procedural protections that may guide HIV control policies. These include the right of a person deprived of liberty to receive reasons for a proposed detention, a fair and independent hearing before an impartial tribunal, and representation for the hearing. Individuals are also entitled to periodic review of the justification for detention (see Chapter 1: Freedom from Arbitrary Arrest, Detention, or Exile).

Detaining people to prevent the spread of HIV is rarely, if ever, necessary and appropriate. In most cases, it substantially burdens human rights and yields little or no public health benefit, because it confines persons who pose minimal risk of infection to others. However, detention may be warranted if an individual intends to harm his or her partner or poses a substantial risk of infecting others. Public officials should determine the risk of infection on a case-by-case basis, since the risk depends largely on behavior which is not amenable to generalizations. Where detention is necessary, the individual has the right to the procedural protections mentioned above. This includes an independent court or tribunal's determination that detention is lawful and periodic review thereafter of the justification (World Health Organization, 1989g).

Statutes, policies, programs, or practices that deprive persons with HIV infection or AIDS of liberty must ensure a minimal level of quality treatment. Persons deprived of liberty for public health purposes are entitled to safe, healthful, and humane conditions and professional medical care. This means that any deprivation of liberty requires a setting and conditions consistent with the purpose of confinement. Persons convicted of criminal offenses must have decent health care, safe and sanitary conditions, proper nutrition, and all appropriate recreational and other privileges within the prison system. This includes, for example, the right not to be placed in seclusion for extended periods and the right to be protected from harm, such as physical violence or infectious disease (e.g., tuberculosis) (see this chapter, Congregate Settings and Institutionalized Persons). The state must place persons confined under public health or mental health powers in appropriate health care facilities suitable to their needs. If persons with HIV infection are subject to isolation, quarantine, or civil commitment, the confinement may not be criminal in nature. Their loss of liberty is not punitive, and they have the right to safe, humane, and healthful conditions (see Chapter 1: Freedom from Inhuman and Degrading Treatment).

States should consider detention, isolation, or quarantine only when it represents the least restrictive alternative that will achieve the public health benefit. In most cases, even policies with coercive elements can include a graded series of alternatives, beginning with voluntary cooperation and incentives. Policymakers should establish specific criteria for employing coercive measures and should compel the use of the least restrictive alternative.

Surveillance

At least twelve countries allow or require authorities to place persons with HIV/AIDS under surveillance (Tomasevski, Gruskin, et al., 1992). Some countries do so under preexisting infectious disease statutes and others do so without legal authorization. Often, civil libertarians and AIDS advocates resist surveillance proposals because they fear the government may control the surveillance or disclose lists of persons with HIV disease (Edgar, Sandomire, 1989).

Individual surveillance differs from epidemiological surveillance, which primarily deals with the distribution, incidence, and prevalence of disease. The proposed public health justification for individual surveillance is that knowing the identity and whereabouts of persons with HIV infection enables authorities to control transmission. This rationale seems logical, but a closer examination suggests otherwise. Mere knowledge of such information, without state action, will not prevent transmission. Monitoring the behavior that may spread HIV infection is highly intrusive and difficult, if not impossible, for the state to observe and record, let alone control.

Surveillance measures burden human rights in several ways. First, monitoring systems, especially those that target intimate behavior, interfere with privacy rights. Breaches of confidentiality concerning HIV status also violate privacy. In addition, where surveillance policies prohibit certain activities, they infringe on freedom of association and expression (see Chapter 1: Privacy; Freedom of Opinion and Expression).

The public health benefits of individual surveillance are minimal and, in most cases, do not justify the substantial human rights burdens. Certain circumstances may present exceptions. For example, a person who had acted dangerously in the past due to physical or mental illness might now be capable of responsible behavior. The state might order community supervision rather than continued detention for such a person. As with all coercive measures, states should employ individual surveillance only where it serves a legitimate purpose, does not cause disproportionate burdens, and represents the least restrictive alternative.

Criminalization

Another response to the HIV/AIDS epidemic is to enact criminal or public health statutes that penalize exposing others to HIV infection. In some cases, states have drafted these laws specifically in response to HIV/AIDS. In others, prosecutors have applied a variety of charges, including assault and attempted murder, to people with HIV infection. States have attempted to punish individuals for potentially transmitting HIV through unprotected sexual intercourse or sharing of drug injection equipment. Some have succeeded in convicting persons for actions that posed an extremely small risk of infection, such as spitting and biting (Gostin, Lazzarini, et al., 1996).

A society's decision to prohibit persons with HIV infection from having sex or sharing needles without informing their partners may be understandable. However, most public health experts question the utility of criminal measures to control the HIV pandemic. Criminalizing HIV transmission is unlikely to have a broad deterrent effect, except, perhaps, for discouraging individuals at risk from seeking testing or services. Additional disadvantages of using criminal penalties for HIV control are that the possibility of prosecution could discourage trust and openness between patients and health care providers and deter some individuals from seeking HIV testing and counseling or any health services.

The criminal approach imposes potentially heavy human rights burdens. States may discriminate in applying such laws, and the stakes are no less than individual liberty and the right to humane treatment (discussed above for isolation and quarantine). Criminal penalties most often target already-marginalized groups, including commercial sex workers, drug users, homosexuals, and prisoners. Punitive laws designed to control disease epidemics harbor an enormous potential for abuse because the police, prosecutors, and jurors exercise considerable discretion. Moreover, a state may target a few publicized individuals and impose penalties in response to deep fears and misunderstandings about HIV and its modes of transmission (Gostin, Lazzarini, et al., 1996b).

Criminal codes can affect persons at risk of HIV infection in a number of ways. States may use existing laws against homosexual activity, prostitution, and drug use to harass persons assumed to be "carriers" of HIV. They may target these groups for arrest, detention, or other official interference on the assumption that removing members of these groups will eliminate the risk of HIV (be it from a neighborhood, city, or country). The structure of a national legal system may (or may not) procedurally protect against unjustified deprivations of liberty. However, the legitimacy of the public health aim in these cases often remains unexamined. For example, the public health goal of a law that punishes only commercial sex workers, and not their clients, for potential HIV transmission is incomplete at best, and, at worst, highly suspect.

Enforcement of criminal laws may directly disrupt AIDS prevention and education efforts. For example, antisodomy laws discourage men from identifying themselves as homosexuals or acknowledging that they have sex with other men. These laws also impede frank discussion of effective prevention methods. Drug paraphernalia laws can have unintended negative public health consequences, such as limiting access to clean injection equipment, criminalizing their possession, or prohibiting needle and syringe exchange programs. Police practices such as using commercial sex workers' possession of condoms as evidence of criminal conduct or criminal intent (see this chapter, Harm Reduction Strategies) may actually increase the risk of spreading HIV if sex workers become unwilling to carry condoms.

Conclusion

How can public health authorities and lawmakers protect both individuals from arbitrary or unnecessary detention and the community? A potential solution is to change the way in which public health authorities define and exercise their powers. To limit the discretionary exercise of power, policymakers should establish criteria defining public health necessity. They should require that any decisions to confine individuals be justified by the best internationally-accepted medical and public health knowledge. Officials should avoid using coercive measures against already-stigmatized groups. Lawmakers should enact graduated series of humane, effective, and minimally restrictive alternatives to protect the community from HIV infection. Finally, legal systems should guarantee that persons deprived of liberty for HIV-related reasons receive full and fair procedural protections proportionate to the burdens on their liberty.

CONGREGATE SETTINGS AND INSTITUTIONALIZED PERSONS

Introduction

HIV infection and AIDS in congregate settings raise serious public health and human rights concerns. This section examines HIV/AIDS control policies for a range of institutionalized persons, including those confined in mental health care institutions, nursing homes, long-term care facilities, migrant worker and refugee camps, prisons, homeless shelters, and the military. After probing the similarities and differences among congregate settings, we closely inspect two settings, prisons and shelter/housing for the homeless. We examine policies designed to control AIDS in these contexts using the Human Rights Impact Assessment.

Public Health and Human Rights in Congregate Settings

Physical, administrative, and institutional characteristics of many congregate settings undermine HIV/AIDS control efforts. These defects do not apply to all congregate living arrangements; indeed, model institutions of every kind exist. Unfortunately, inappropriate practices, limited resources, and inattention from health policymakers often combine to produce serious problems.

Similarities among congregate settings

An institution's physical characteristics can profoundly affect the health of residents in congregate settings. Crowding and poor ventilation facilitate transmission of airborne diseases like tuberculosis. Inadequate sanitary facilities, infrequent access to clean water, and low hygiene standards lead to outbreaks of diarrheal disease. Malnutrition among residents, because of either preexisting conditions (homelessness or refugee status) or inadequate, unhealthy institutional food, increases their susceptibility to disease and severe malnutrition. The presence of residents who are immunocompromised due to HIV or other diseases increases the risk of rapid transmission and widespread illness. One of the earliest-documented clusters of multi-drug resistant tuberculosis (MDR-TB) transmission in the United States occurred among residents of a long-term care facility for persons with HIV (Centers for Disease Control and Prevention, 1991). Dozens of other outbreaks of MDR-TB in hospitals, shelters, and prisons have disproportionately affected persons with HIV infection or AIDS.

Public health problems stem from the traditional characteristics of institutional settings. Inadequate supervision, poor security, and minimal privacy are features of unsafe environments in which assault, rape, and drug use are constant dangers. Camps for refugees or displaced persons are often unsafe due to the threat of conflict, disaster, or aggression. Camps may actually expose residents to substantial physical and mental harm. At the site of what was formerly the largest camp for displaced persons on the Thai border with Cambodia, seven percent of the residents identified the most terrible event in their lives as occurring during the last year *while they lived in the camp*, worse even than living under the Khmer Rouge regime in Cambodia, from which they fled (Mollica, Donelan, et al., 1991). Similarly, domestic prisons often expose inmates to greater violence than they experience before confinement. Commentators suggest that some correctional authorities are unable to prevent sexual aggression among prisoners because of crowding and inadequate supervision (Hammett, 1987).

A recent American court decision ordered the closure of the detention center at Guantanamo Bay, Cuba, calling it an "HIV prison camp." The camp was established to detain HIV-infected refugees from Haiti who sought political asylum in the United States. The court found that "the Haitians' plight is a tragedy of immense proportion" based on the inadequate medical care, housing, and legal representation there (Tabor, 1993). President Clinton subsequently disbanded the camp and permitted entry of the political asylees into the United States.

Institutional administrators and private parties who deal with persons in congregate settings frequently have objectives that supersede health care, health education, and even disease control. The administrators of institutions for mentally ill or retarded persons may focus on controlling residents' behavior and providing for their basic bodily needs rather than screening or preventing communicable diseases through health education or prevention measures. Military or security officials may value troop discipline and readiness over respect for autonomy or confidentiality. Camps for migrant workers may supply employers with ready sources of inexpensive agricultural, construction, or manufacturing labor; without benefits such as health care or a healthy environment in which to live, residents may have poor access to acute care, preventive care, health education, and substance abuse treatment.

Finally, the issue of vulnerability underlies each congregate setting. Persons living in these settings (with the possible exception of the military) tend to have low status in society—homeless persons, mentally ill or retarded persons, prisoners, refugees, displaced persons, children who are wards of the state, and persons requiring long-term care. Many of these groups are disproportionately affected by HIV/AIDS. Members of these groups lack strong advocates and often suffer discrimination because of their status. Instead of receiving the greatest protection, the most vulnerable members of society frequently receive the least.

Differences among congregate settings

Differences exist among congregate settings—in mission, population, locus of control, and daily administration. Furthermore, national and regional variations may arise from different social, cultural, or religious foundations or from different levels of resources and economic development. Perhaps the most obvious distinction among the types of congregate settings is the degree of control that authorities exercise over the residents. In some settings, such as homeless shelters or migrant worker camps, the residents may come and go with relative freedom; in others, such as prisons or mental institutions, residents do not have that option. Freedom of movement within the institution also varies widely. Many camps for refugees or displaced persons function like self-contained cities in which trade, education, and family affairs (including births, marriages, and funerals) occur without supervision. On the other hand, maximum security prisons may hold inmates in their cells twenty-three hours a day or impose periods of complete isolation.

The potential for HIV transmission varies with the setting, the extent of authoritative control, and the residents' level of seroprevalence and risk-taking behavior. Persons in institutions where drug use and sexual activity occur frequently are at heightened risk through different routes of transmission. Prisons or homeless shelters with many injecting drug users (IDUs) are likely to have higher transmission rates than those serving elderly, severely disabled, mentally ill, or retarded persons. Prisons and other sex-segregated institutions have a greater potential for homosexual contact than do nonsegregated settings (where heterosexual transmission may be the primary route). Any institution for women of child-bearing age who have HIV infection harbors the potential for perinatal transmission. Discerning the potential for and likely modes of transmission is crucial in designing and implementing sound HIV prevention and control policies.

In introducing HIV prevention strategies, authorities sometimes cite the unusual nature of their institutions and the special health risks involved. In the United States, military authorities justify mandatory HIV testing on two grounds: to exclude HIV-infected recruits and to reassign HIV-infected active duty personnel. The first is purported to protect the blood supply, since combat units serve as their own blood banks while in the field. The second is claimed to safeguard HIV-infected soldiers from the infectious and opportunistic diseases to which they may be exposed during overseas assignments.

Government and institutional authorities from a variety of congregate settings adopt many of the same public health policies and programs. An examination of two settings, prisons and shelters for the homeless, illustrates that these programs possess profound public health policy and human rights implications.

Prisons

Public health measures frequently target prisons to control HIV/AIDS. Most studies of seroprevalence among prisoners indicate that they are more likely than the general population to have HIV infection. The reasons for this vary with region and from industrialized to developing countries. In specific southern European countries, high seroprevalence among prisoners (Spain, 26% and Italy, 17%) may be attributed to high rates of injecting drug use among prisoners prior to their incarceration and high levels of infection among IDUs in those countries (Harding, 1987). In some developing countries, AIDS cases among prisoners reflect the predominance of young adults in the prison population—the same age group with the highest seroprevalence due to heterosexual transmission (Chambuso, 1991). Certain behaviors that occur in prisons, such as injection drug use and homosexual activity, are common modes of transmission. Studies of transmission among inmates, however, have been inconclusive, sometimes suggesting rather low rates (Hammett, 1989). Regardless of the evidence on transmission within prison, authorities should be concerned about the many ramifications of HIV disease. In many countries, HIV has exposed the inadequacies of prison health care (Thomas, Costigan, 1992). Moreover, prisons are not static environments; most prisoners move back (and forth) to the surrounding community after a relatively short period of time. Consequently, HIV-prevention efforts in prisons (or the lack thereof) also impact the risk of infection for families and communities.

Most public health measures to prevent the spread of HIV in prisons have focused on screening or segregating infected prisoners (Tomasevski, Gruskin, et al., 1992). A study commissioned by the Council of Europe in 1986 found that four out of seventeen countries had compulsory testing policies for prisoners, and seven countries segregated HIV-infected prisoners in housing or work activities (Harding, Schaller, 1992). The federal prison system in the United States and at least sixteen of its state systems have policies of compulsory screening; fewer employ segregation (Andrus, Fleming, et al., 1989). National courts have tended to permit prison authorities broad discretion in screening and segregating individuals and have upheld challenged programs (Gostin, Lazzarini, et al., 1996b; Gostin, 1989, 1990a). Prison policies may also concern prevention and education, access to harm reduction strategies, and medical research involving prisoners. Some policies may be discriminatory in that they treat prisoners differently, based solely on HIV infection, and without valid public health or security justifications. We briefly examine each type.

Screening

Compulsory screening in the absence of other effective policies is unlikely to protect inmates' health. Screening will not detect all HIV-infected prisoners in any system, due to delayed seroconversion and the potential for false negatives. Nor has data shown that performance of the test alone, or knowledge of the test result, without counseling, changes subsequent behavior. Compulsory screening without concomitant counseling or education neglects one of the most effective aspects of prevention: the opportunity to explain and discuss the import and consequences of the HIV test. Screening might also have a negative public health impact if it creates a false sense of security and therefore promotes risk-taking among prisoners who believe they are not infected.

Compulsory HIV screening of institutionalized populations significantly burdens their human rights. That prisoners are lawfully detained does not mean that they forgo all human rights. Prisoners retain the right to refuse testing or treatment, the right to privacy, the right to be treated with dignity, and the right to decide for themselves about medical intervention. No justification exists for compulsory testing of a prisoner unless she receives HIV education and counseling and does not engage in high-risk behavior. The World Health Organization describes the compulsory testing of prisoners as "unethical and ineffective" and calls for its prohibition (World Health Organization, 1993b).

Voluntary testing and counseling for HIV infection form an important part of HIV prevention programs in prison. Effective policies that also respect human rights include providing inmates access to voluntary testing as part of a broader education and counseling effort, and testing where clinically indicated as part of comprehensive health care. Prisons can and should safeguard HIV-related information as part of their screening, testing, medical care, and information storage policies (see this chapter, Epidemiological Surveillance and Disease Control).

Segregation or isolation of HIV-infected prisoners

Segregation, special confinement, or other restrictions, based on HIV status alone, may constitute unjustified discrimination. Such policies deny prisoners the limited liberties enjoyed by inmates incarcerated for similar offenses and with similar records of conduct. Most importantly, segregation and isolation policies based solely on an inmate's HIV status are unnecessary and ineffective means by which to control HIV in prisons (World Health Organization, 1993b). Segregation policies are overinclusive where they confine all prisoners with HIV infection, regardless of behavior. Only those prisoners who place others at risk merit isolation or segregation. Segregation strategies are underinclusive where authorities arbitrarily implement them. For example, confining only HIV-infected persons who seek testing, or those who have advanced disease, likely excludes some inmates who pose an equal or greater public health danger, and it may increase risk-taking among nonsegregated prisoners.

Establishing "AIDS units" in prisons effectively discloses the inmates' HIV infection to the entire prison population and community. This breach of confidentiality exposes segregated inmates to discrimination, ostracism, and perhaps even violence. Upon release, these individuals may face discrimination or rejection by employers, landlords, and community or family members.

Segregation policies highlight the larger issue of what constitutes an acceptable standard of care for prisoners infected with HIV. Separate confinement often entails inferior living conditions, exposure to other infectious diseases, and little (if any) access to recreation, association, work, or religious observance within the prison community. At the Wandsworth prison in Great Britain, authorities kept HIV-infected prisoners and those awaiting test results in a "small, dingy and airless basement" (Thomas, Costigan, 1992). Authorities restricted the inmates' access to exercise and classes and even denied them the use of bath or shower facilities. Such confinement could impair both physical and mental health, especially for prisoners serving long sentences or those with advanced HIV disease. One court in the United States ordered corrections officials to build well-ventilated facilities for HIV-infected inmates.

Although prison authorities commonly have considerable discretion in determining the conditions of confinement, international human rights norms establish basic standards. International instruments such as the Standard Minimum Rules for the Treatment of Prisoners and the Convention Against Torture, and Other Cruel, Inhuman or Degrading Treatment or Punishment require that prisoners live in adequate conditions of confinement and treatment. Segregating or isolating HIV-infected prisoners in substandard conditions may violate prisoners' rights to be free from cruel, inhuman, or degrading treatment. The European Committee on the Prevention of Torture and Inhuman or Degrading Treatment has condemned segregation in the United Kingdom and the "impoverished environment" in which HIV-infected prisoners were held (*Lancet* editorial, 1991). In addition, the United States National Commission on AIDS has concluded that much treatment of prisoners with AIDS has been "cruel and unusual" (1990).

Humane and dignified treatment and health care

Prisoners and their advocates claim the right to humane and dignified treatment within the prison system and upon release. International jurisprudence in the area of mental health suggests that such a right exists and that very poor conditions may violate it (see Chapter 1: Freedom From Inhuman and Degrading Treatment). The Human Rights Committee has interpreted the right to humane treatment as a "basic standard of universal application which cannot depend entirely on material resources" (Human Rights Committee).

In the context of HIV control, humane and dignified treatment of prisoners includes more than safe and healthful living conditions. It requires access to medical care, drug treatment, and special services for HIV-infected prisoners, and provisions for compassionate release or transfer to a hospital or hospice for persons dying of AIDS (World Health Organization, 1993b). Moreover, the "equivalence principle" of health care suggests that prisoners with HIV disease deserve at least the same level of health care as is available outside the prison (Thomas, Costigan, 1992). The European Prison Rules embody this principle, and the British Medical Association and others support it. Similarly, the WHO recommends that prisoners have access to the same level of specialized care for AIDS and HIV-related illnesses as do members of the surrounding community (1987e, 1993b).

Women, who make up a minority of the prison population in most countries, have additional specialized needs which authorities routinely fail to address. Like men, women inmates have higher rates of HIV infection than the general population. In industrialized countries, this may be because many female inmates are IDUs, partners of IDUs, or commercial sex workers. In developing countries, HIV infection among women prisoners may reflect high rates of infection among young adults, who comprise the majority of prison populations. Humane and dignified treatment for women prisoners includes gynecological treatment, education on safer sex practices and mother-to-child transmission, counseling, obstetrical care for pregnant prisoners, and access to abortion for women wishing to terminate a pregnancy. Treatment should also include medical care for children born to HIV-infected women and opportunities for women to care for their very young children while incarcerated (World Health Organization, 1993b; Harding, Schaller, 1992).

Given scarce resources, states may consider denying HIV services to inmates rather than to law-abiding citizens. But failing to meet minimal standards for imprisonment conditions and health care violates international human rights law. Moreover, such a decision may undermine the state's own interests. Since many incarcerations are relatively short-term, preventing HIV transmission in prison is an investment in the public health of the broader community. For example, education and counseling programs in prisons may effect behavioral changes that continue upon the individual's release (see this chapter, Prevention and Education). Providing gynecological and prenatal care to women prisoners may improve the health of both mothers and newborns and reduce their future reliance on the state. Identifying inmates with HIV infection (through voluntary testing) and treating them prophylactically for opportunistic infections, such as TB, may prevent the spread of these diseases within the prison and the community.

Part of governments' obligation to provide humane and dignified treatment is to protect persons who depend on the state from communicable diseases and violence by guards and other inmates. Outbreaks of active TB among prisoners and staff have been documented in western Europe and the United States. This problem (although perhaps unrecognized) likely exists in developing countries where TB is endemic (Harding, Schaller, 1992). Since co-infection with TB and HIV promotes the rapid spread of TB, HIV control policies in prisons should prioritize control of communicable diseases, including TB (World Health Organization, 1993b).

The growing global awareness of the danger of HIV infection has drawn attention to the poor security and conditions in many prisons. State action is sorely needed to prevent the coercion of inmates into sex through intimidation or physical or sexual assault. States should reduce crowding, improve the level and quality of security and supervision, and ensure opportunities for safe, healthful activities. Coercive measures, such as segregation of aggressive inmates (whether HIV-infected or not), may be a necessary last resort to protect other inmates and staff (World Health Organization, 1993b).

Discriminatory policies

According to a United Nations (1991) special report, many countries have reported discriminatory policies and practices by prison administrators against prisoners infected with HIV. These have included compulsory testing and isolation, denial of medical care, subjection to human rights abuses, degrading treatment, and harassment.

Specialists convened by the WHO (1987e, 1993b) recommended that states should not subject prisoners to discriminatory measures on the basis of HIV infection except where required for the prisoner's own health. Strategies such as involuntary testing, segregation, and isolation do not promote this goal. Limiting opportunities of HIV-infected prisoners to work, education, religious observance, and visits from family and friends are needlessly discriminatory in most circumstances. Unnecessary special precautions, such as staff's use of gloves or masks whenever touching or accompanying HIV-infected prisoners, also stigmatize and discriminate against them.

Although states may lawfully limit it, liberty remains fundamental to human dignity. AIDS control policies severely restrict liberty when they constrict freedom of movement within closed environments and impede access to services, recreation, or work assignments. Given the lack of evidence of casual HIV transmission, such intrusions are usually unnecessary from a public health perspective and needlessly stigmatize and dehumanize prisoners with HIV disease. States must appropriately justify added limitations on institutionalized persons' liberty by objective, nondiscriminatory criteria and as the least restrictive alternative (see Chapter 1: Nondiscrimination; Freedom from Arbitrary Arrest, Detention, or Exile).

Prevention and education

The HIV/AIDS pandemic has forced public health, prison, and government authorities to acknowledge that sexual activity and drug use occur in prisons even where both are strictly forbidden. Persons incarcerated against their will are particularly dependent on the state for information, education, and the means to prevent HIV transmission. For this reason, the WHO (1987e, 1993b) has recommended that states provide comprehensive education and prevention programs for prison inmates and staff and consider providing condoms and sterile injection equipment within prisons. The Council of Europe (1988) has gone further by advocating the supply of condoms, and as a "last resort," clean, single-use syringes and needles in prisons. In practice, condom distribution has gained wider acceptance than the needle proposal. A WHO study found that twenty-three of fifty-two national prison systems sampled permit condom distribution while none authorize distribution of clean injection equipment (Harding, Schaller, 1992). By the mid-1990s, some European prison officials had broadened HIV prevention efforts to address syringe-related transmission. In 1996, Swiss researchers reported on a pilot project that included a syringe exchange program in a women's prison in Bern (Zeegers Paget, Bernasconi, et al., 1996).

Research

Medical researchers have long used institutionalized persons as subjects. These persons make convenient research populations, in part because they are located in one place, facilitating follow-up. Historically, researchers and prison authorities have loosely applied or altogether ignored the principles of informed consent.

The Nuremberg Code (1947), the Declaration of Helsinki (World Medical Association, 1964), resolutions of the Council of Europe (1990), and the Council of International Organizations of Medical Sciences (1991, 1993) require the express informed consent of all subjects who participate in biomedical or epidemiologic research. These documents provide added protections to those who are unable to give informed consent (e.g., children and mentally incompetent persons). Importantly, they recommend special protections for research on confined populations and the military. These populations may be pressured to consent to research. Accordingly, ethical reviews of research on institutionalized populations must ensure that no undue inducements are offered to participate in research, and that a significant opportunity exists to benefit the individual and the population. As efforts to develop and test candidate vaccines and drugs for HIV infection advance, society must safeguard institutionalized populations from exploitation (For more discussion, see this chapter, Research on Human Subjects: International Ethical Guidelines).

Homeless Shelters or Housing

Homelessness and substandard housing is a growing problem worldwide. The figures are staggering; more than one billion people in developed and developing countries lack adequate housing (Hendriks, Leckie, 1991). The Council of Europe estimates that approximately ten million people in Europe have inadequate housing (Hendriks, 1992). Many developing countries have recently undergone rapid urbanization, in which large numbers of the rural poor migrate to "megacities" in search of jobs. Many of these workers and their families lack housing; others live in shantytowns without clean water, sewage systems, or electricity.

People who do not have homes are particularly vulnerable to HIV disease and associated infections, such as tuberculosis. Most are malnourished, are in generally poor health, and are unlikely to have the means or the ability to protect themselves from HIV infection by always using condoms or clean injection equipment. Many have limited access to medical care or health education. A study in San Francisco found that homeless adults had rates of HIV infection ten times that of people with homes (*San Francisco Chronicle*, 1991). New York alone has at least 8,000 homeless people with AIDS (Cohen, Weiseberg, 1990). Furthermore, these persons may be poorly equipped to avoid infection due to mental illness, addiction, or prostitution (in exchange for food, money, or drugs). Those with mental illnesses may be especially susceptible to sexual exploitation and substance abuse (Susser, Valencia, et al., 1993). HIV infection is a particular peril for the increasing numbers of homeless children throughout the world. Child prostitution, sexual abuse, and drug use among "street children" can all lead to HIV infection in adolescence (Koopman, Rosario, et al., 1994).

Tragically, being diagnosed with HIV disease may itself lead to homelessness. Because of irrational fears, landlords, neighbors, or families may deny persons with HIV infection or AIDS access to public housing, evict them from private housing, or banish them from their homes (Hendriks, 1992). Nursing homes and other long-term care facilities have rejected AIDS patients who are too ill to live independently. Organizations seeking to help AIDS patients have been denied permits or leases for hospices or have encountered bitter community opposition (United Nations, 1991).

The last two decades have seen a growing acceptance of the right to adequate shelter or housing as a basic human right (Leckie, 1992; Hendriks, Leckie, 1991; see Chapter 1: The Right to an Adequate Standard of Living, Including Food and Shelter). More than thirty countries have constitutionally guaranteed housing to every citizen, regardless of health status (Leckie, 1992). However, realization of this right lags far behind its theoretical acceptance. Where a government undertakes to provide shelter, particularly to a vulnerable population, it is obliged to maintain a minimum level of safety and health. All levels of government antidiscrimination policies help prevent persons from losing their homes.

The problems of homelessness and substandard housing are daunting tasks for many governments. Some of the adopted solutions have serious public health or human rights failings. In industrialized countries, for instance, large, crowded shelters with poor security may leave residents vulnerable to intimidation, physical or sexual assault, and robbery. Old buildings with poor ventilation and crowding invite the spread of TB and other communicable diseases. The anonymity and limited resources of shelter systems result in haphazard health care for people without homes. Some homeless persons avoid shelters because they perceive them as dangerous places.

Public health authorities seeking to protect the health of homeless people face a challenge. Many homeless people want and need protection from the weather, violent crime, and communicable diseases. If public health measures are primarily "medical" and involve coercion (such as compulsory screening, isolation, or segregation), they risk driving homeless persons away from the settings intended to help them. Such public health measures overlook some of the underlying causes of homeless persons' vulnerability to HIV infection (e.g., injection drug or other substance abuse, sexual exploitation, and mental illness). To illustrate, tuberculosis control measures that have focused exclusively on "medical interventions" such as screening, detection of active disease, and isolation during the infectious stage have often failed. Many homeless TB patients, released from acute care hospitals to the streets, fail to complete treatment and relapse into active disease. Sometimes reactivated TB becomes resistant to standard treatments, leading to dangerous increases in multi-drug resistant TB (MDR-TB) among the homeless (Neville,

Bromberg, et al., 1994). More successful programs have combined medical interventions with supervised treatment and access to social services (Frieden, Fujiwara, et al., 1995; Gostin, Lazzarini, 1994). HIV prevention and care policies for homeless persons should be comprehensive and well tailored to their needs. Ideally, a state would provide education about HIV, access to preventive measures, drug treatment, medical care, long-term housing, and, where suitable, vocational training or education.

HARM REDUCTION STRATEGIES: STERILE DRUG INJECTION EQUIPMENT AND CONDOMS

Introduction

Few issues at the intersection of public health and human rights are as fraught with conflict as harm reduction strategies. These approaches recognize that many individuals will not abstain from drugs or sex but may behave more safely if armed with education, counseling, and the means to protect themselves. These strategies take many forms. This chapter focuses on the distribution or exchange of sterile injection equipment, bleach programs, and the distribution of condoms.

Harm reduction strategies most effectively achieve public health goals and are most accepted by communities when they are part of a comprehensive prevention and education program. Integrating such strategies into other efforts—to educate and empower individuals and communities, and to ensure access to drug treatment, health care, social services, and job training—improves their efficacy (see this chapter, Prevention and Education).

Two main harm reduction strategies for HIV involve distributing clean drug injection equipment and condoms. Ideally, programs that offer sterile injection equipment to IDUs also relay the importance of practicing safer sex. Many existing programs provide sterile equipment, bleach for decontamination of used equipment, and condoms in kits (Centers for Disease Control and Prevention, 1995d; World Health Organization Global Programme on AIDS, 1991a).

Despite their public health advantages, harm reduction strategies often arouse substantial opposition. In some communities, parents and religious leaders object to such programs because of the perception that they will promote premarital or extramarital sexual activity and/or drug use. Opponents also argue that harm reduction programs targeted toward young people interfere with parents' rights to direct their children's education. Some view these programs as sanctioning dangerous, unlawful, or immoral behavior. Thus, differences of opinion on both human rights and public health exist. Empirical evidence may help to resolve this conflict. We should ask: (1) Do harm reduction programs increase sex or drug use? and (2) Do they effectively reduce the prevalence of HIV, STIs, unwanted pregnancies, and drug use?

Distribution or Exchange of Sterile Injection Equipment

Background

Sharing drug injection equipment is one of the primary routes of HIV transmission in many parts of Europe and North and South America. By the end of 1994, approximately one-third of AIDS cases reported in the United States were attributable to injecting drug use (Centers for Disease Control and Prevention, 1995e). Parts of Eastern Europe and Southeast Asia have also experienced a rapid increase in HIV seroprevalence among injecting drug users (IDUs) in these regions (Stimson, Hunter, et al., 1996; Porter, Gostin, 1992). Studies of IDUs have identified strong social and cultural forces underlying this practice. Sharing drug injection equipment can be a form of social bonding or camaraderie among sexual partners, friends, or other users in a shooting gallery (Des Jarlais, Friedman, 1988). Recent research suggests that sharing is also directly correlated with a limited supply of needles and syringes; where drug users cannot legally obtain or possess new injection equipment, they are more likely to share or reuse syringes and less likely to maintain safer injection practices. (Koester, 1994; Nelson, Vlahov, et al., 1991).

The WHO's Global Programme on AIDS (1988c) consensus report on HIV and drug use set out three broad strategies to combat the spread of HIV among IDUs: education, drug treatment, and access to sterile injection equipment. Consequently, in addition to educational efforts to change the social behaviors and rituals that lead to sharing, many public health officials have attempted to make sterile equipment more available.

More than thirty countries have facilitated IDUs' access to sterile injection equipment as part of their HIV prevention strategy. Exchange programs originally began in the Netherlands to reduce the spread of hepatitis B among hard-to-reach IDUs (Hartgers, Buning, et al., 1989; van den Hoek, van Haastrecht, et al., 1989). Countries following suit include Australia (Wodak, Dolan, et al., 1987; Wolk, Wodak, et al., 1990), Canada (Bardsley, Turvey, et al., 1990), Sweden (Ljungberg, Christensson, et al., 1991), the United Kingdom (Donoghoe, Stimson, et al., 1989; Stimson, Alldritt, et al., 1988), and others.

These programs vary by content and sponsor. The government, private organizations, and IDUs or former IDUs may operate distributions or exchanges of sterile equipment. Public policy may abet access by relaxing legal requirements that pharmacies sell equipment only by prescription; or by permitting sales through vending machines or locations other than pharmacies. In much of the world, unrestricted sale of injection equipment has been the norm. Convincing IDUs, especially those in developing countries, to use sterile equipment, however, may require specially targeted education efforts and/or measures to make sterile equipment affordable (Choopanya, Vanichiseni, et al., 1991). In relatively wealthy countries, simply allowing sale through pharmacies can significantly reduce sharing among IDUs and can decrease IDUs' procurement of syringes from unsafe sources (e.g., street sellers) (Groseclose, Weinstein, et al., 1995). In addition, drug treatment to eliminate IDUs' dependence on drugs or to allow them to satisfy their craving through oral means can constitute part of a comprehensive harm reduction strategy. Methadone programs, which replace use of injection drugs with oral doses of methadone, have attracted renewed interest.

Goals of needle and syringe distribution or exchange programs

Harm reduction strategies for IDUs have several objectives: (1) to decrease the incidence of blood-borne diseases including HIV and hepatitis B; (2) to reduce the use of injection drugs by bringing more IDUs into treatment through education, referrals, and access to social services; (3) to encourage IDUs already infected with HIV to obtain needed clinical care, as well as counseling and education; and (4) to remove contaminated injection equipment from circulation.

Advantages and disadvantages in practice

The ability of exchange or distribution programs to reduce rates of HIV transmission is difficult to measure because of the long incubation period of HIV, the challenge of following IDUs over time, the human rights implications of HIV-antibody screening, and the expense and methodological complications of designing reliable studies (Normand, Vlahov, et al., 1995; Stryker, Smith, 1993).

Despite these obstacles, increasing evidence suggests that harm reduction strategies achieve compelling public health objectives. A correlation seems to exist between adopting such strategies and slowing the HIV seroprevalence rate among IDUs. Some jurisdictions that restrict the sale or possession of injection equipment have high HIV seroprevalence among IDUs (Edinburgh, thirty-eight to sixty-eight percent and New York, fifty to sixty percent). Conversely, other jurisdictions with fewer restrictions report lower HIV seroprevalence among IDUs (Glasgow, 4.5 percent and Amsterdam 3.4 percent; Joseph, Des Jarlais, 1989). In addition, jurisdictions with established exchange or distribution programs have seen the seroprevalence rate slow among IDUs (Wood, 1990). Although the data do not establish a causal link between limits on sterile injection equipment and the HIV seroprevalence rate, they suggest that supply limitations do not decrease seroprevalence rates; rather, readily accessible supplies may slow increases in HIV seroprevalence (Gostin, 1991b).

A model developed at Yale University to estimate the impact of a needle exchange program on HIV transmission among program participants in New Haven, Connecticut, suggests that such programs are effective. The model predicts a thirty-three percent reduction in new HIV infections over one year among program participants. The underlying theory is that by exchanging unused needles in return for used ones, the program may reduce the period during which needles circulate, thus reducing the opportunity for contamination, sharing, and HIV transmission (United States General Accounting Office, 1993).

Studies of needle exchange programs document their achievement of more immediate goals: (1) reducing the incidence of needle sharing, the prevalence of injection drug use, and the frequency of injection; (2) promoting the safe disposal of contaminated needles; and (3) serving as a bridge to treatment (United States General Accounting Office, 1993).

Reducing the occurrence of shared contaminated injection equipment reduces the risk of IDUs contracting HIV infection; several studies show that IDUs who enter syringe exchange programs share equipment less. Data indicate that the longer an IDU attends exchange programs, the more likely he or she is to report significant reductions in sharing behavior (New York City Department of Health, 1989; Hartgers, Buning, et al., 1989; Hagan, Des Jarlais, et al., 1991). Moreover, the longer the client participates, the more likely he or she is to rely exclusively on the exchange program as his or her source of injection equipment (van den Hoek, van Haastrecht, et al., 1989). However, an English study found that regular attendees of an exchange program were more likely to lend injection equipment due to pressure to supply other IDUs with sterile equipment (Klee, Faugier, et al., 1991). Evidence of reduced sharing suggests that drug users are becoming more aware of the risks of HIV, more concerned about their health, and more willing to alter their behavior to avoid blood-borne infections (Des Jarlais, Friedman, 1988; Centers for Disease Control and Prevention, 1990).

In recent years, panels of experts have studied whether needle and syringe exchange and other measures that increase access to sterile injection equipment prevent HIV infection. Although no definitive evidence exists of the efficacy of syringe exchange programs in reducing HIV and other blood-borne pathogens among IDUs, researchers are cautiously optimistic about the benefits of syringe exchange programs, and they support governments' endorsement of these strategies as part of a comprehensive HIV prevention effort (Normand, Vlahov, et al., 1995; Lurie, Reingold, et al., 1993).

Exchange programs have an important advantage over distribution programs in that they reduce the number of contaminated needles in circulation. Data from a Netherlands program found that needle return increased from seventy percent to ninety-five percent over three years (San Francisco AIDS Foundation, 1989).

Perhaps the most promising aspect of the various studies is the potential for needle and syringe exchanges to link IDUs to drug as well as STI and TB treatment. Drug users usually have pressing health and welfare needs but are notoriously difficult to reach. Offering these persons a service facilitates positive contact. Considerable public health gains may result from needle and syringe exchanges that offer drug users HIV testing, counseling, sex education, treatment referrals, housing, and social support. Needle and syringe exchange programs in Tacoma, Washington (Hagan, Des Jarlais, et al., 1991), New York City (New York City Department of Health, 1989), Sweden (Ljungberg, Christensonn, et al., 1991) and Vancouver (Bardsley, Turvey, et al., 1990) report that significant numbers of previously untreated drug users have been referred for drug treatment and other services. In New Haven, Connecticut, syringe exchange program operators noted that even IDUs who did not use the exchange to obtain injection equipment often stopped by for drug treatment information (Heimer, 1994).

Residents of poor inner-city areas sometimes view these distribution programs as the state's overly simplistic solution to a complex problem—that is, a way to abandon communities that the authorities are unable or unwilling to protect from the violence and crime associated with the drug trade. This has led some communities to accuse policymakers of discrimination and even attempted genocide against inner-city minority populations (Marriott, 1988). Some members of these communities assert that they should have the right to determine the priorities for public health interventions that affect them; they might allocate resources to eliminate drug use rather than to combat AIDS (Dalton, 1989).

Cost is another issue for public health officials to consider in designing HIV prevention programs in an area with limited resources. Needle and syringe exchanges require an investment of resources (e.g., personnel, supplies, buildings, or vehicles). The estimated cost of operating a syringe exchange program per HIV infection prevented ranges from $3,700 to $12,000 (U.S.) (Lurie, Reingold, et al., 1993; Normand, Vlahov, et al., 1995). Although this figure is far below the estimated lifetime cost of HIV-associated medical costs ($119,000 U.S.) (Hellinger, 1993), communities may be unwilling or unable to invest this amount in a syringe exchange program. Policymakers, however, can increase access to needles and syringes with little or no investment of public resources by repealing or reforming laws that limit access to sterile injection equipment. Where this has been tried in the United States, the first-year results show a nearly forty percent decrease in self-reported sharing among IDUs and a shift in the primary source of syringes from "street sellers" to pharmacies (Groseclose, Weinstein, et al., 1995).

For communities suffering from the dual epidemics of drug dependency and HIV, a crucial issue is whether harm reduction programs (syringe distribution, exchange, or legalized sale) encourage or facilitate drug use. Several needle and syringe exchange projects have found no increases in drug use and less injecting by IDU participants (van den Hoek, van Haastrecht, et al., 1989; Hagan, Des Jarlais, et al., 1991; Hartgers, Buning, et al., 1989; Hart, Carvell, et al., 1989; Wolk, Wodak, et al., 1990). No findings demonstrate that syringe distribution or exchange increases first use or greater use of injection drugs among IDUs (Watters, Cheng, et al., 1991). Two major reviews of studies of syringe exchange programs in the United States and abroad concluded that no evidence suggested that programs increased use or encouraged new users (Normand, Vlahov, et al., 1995; Lurie, Reingold, et al., 1993). These data and the conclusions of experts may assuage local communities' concerns about the "mixed messages" presented by such projects. Project sponsors must be sensitive and respectful of community cultures, morals, and beliefs. Exchange programs must be integrated with an array of services designed to combat the drug epidemic, the associated violence, and the spread of HIV.

Legal barriers to needle and syringe distribution and exchange

In many countries, laws prohibit needle distribution or exchange programs. The most common barrier is drug paraphernalia laws. These laws make selling, distributing, or possessing equipment for the purpose of using illicit drugs a criminal offense. Drug paraphernalia laws usually do not prohibit over-the-counter sale of syringes and needles by pharmacists. Instead, they criminalize the sale, distribution, possession, manufacture, or advertising of equipment intended for use with illegal drugs. A second, less common legal bar are needle prescription laws. Such laws, usually coexisting with drug paraphernalia statutes, ban the sale, distribution, or possession of syringes and needles without a medical prescription. In jurisdictions with these laws, pharmacists need a valid prescription by a licensed medical doctor to be authorized to sell injection equipment (Gostin, Lazzarini, et al., 1996b; Porter, Gostin, 1992). On several occasions, the United States Congress has specifically prohibited or restricted the use of federal funds to support needle exchange programs. Since 1988, Congress has passed at least eight statutes that contain provisions prohibiting or restricting the use of federal funds for syringe exchange programs and activities (Office of the General Counsel, 1994; United States General Accounting Office, 1993).

Community leaders (e.g., *Spokane County Health District v. Brockett*, 120 Wash. 2d 140 [1992]) and public health departments (e.g., *Commonwealth v. Leno*, 415 Mass. 835 [1993]) in the United States have litigated to obtain the right to operate exchange projects. Their claims have invoked the public health exigency that prompted the exchanges and the "public health necessity" defense. In some cases, public health officials and community activists have succeeded (Gostin, 1993; *Spokane County Health District v. Brockett*, 1992; *People v. Bordowitz*, 588 N.Y.S.2d 507 [1991]). Other courts have upheld convictions of syringe exchange personnel, refusing to allow defendants to argue medical necessity to justify violating syringe laws (*Commonwealth v. Leno*, 1993; *State v. Sorge*, 591 A.2d 1382 [1991]).

Public health officials, law enforcement officials, and community leaders must harmonize their objectives and cooperate in combatting the dual epidemics of drug dependency and HIV. Nothing could be more destructive of public health goals than to disseminate clean needles and syringes and then arrest the user for possessing drug paraphernalia or for violating prescription laws and regulations. Where drug control and public health policies work in concert, perhaps even synergistically, the population benefits from both a human rights and a public health perspective.

Human rights implications of failing to provide adequate means for safer injection of drugs

Failure to build harm reduction strategies into prevention programs burdens human rights. Individuals have the right to be fully informed and educated about the health risks of syringe sharing and unprotected sex (UDHR, Art. 26.1, 26.2; ICESCR, Art. 13.1). Individuals also have the right to seek, exchange, and impart information freely, even if doing so offends others (UDHR, Art. 19; ICCPR, Art. 19). The rights to education and information can form the foundation for enjoyment of the right to health and, ultimately, to life (For a more detailed examination of these rights, see this chapter, Prevention and

Education, and Chapter 1: The Right to Health; Right to Life; The Right to Education; Freedom of Opinion and Expression). Governmental failure to inform people of the significance of and to increase access to sterile injection equipment may burden the rights to education, health, and life.

Programs that provide sterile injection equipment to IDUs often face apparently conflicting tasks. They must reach a population sorely in need of the information and of the means to protect themselves from HIV infection. At the same time, they must respond to concerns that outsiders will force programs upon the community that will exacerbate the drug problem. Involving community members and IDUs in decisions about HIV prevention efforts from the outset may promote understanding and cooperation. Failure to gain the acceptance of non-IDUs will undermine the public health program, as will failure to earn IDUs' trust. Syringe exchange programs should be part of a comprehensive package of services, including education, increased access to high-quality drug treatment, and health care, that seek to interrupt and end the cycle of poverty, drug use, and AIDS (Gostin, Lazzarini, et al., 1996b; Gostin, 1991b). Syringe exchange programs will be most effective as part of a comprehensive public health effort aimed at reducing drug dependency and blood-borne diseases among IDUs. They will also be more acceptable to IDUs, the community, and society burdened by HIV infection and injection drug use.

Providing Information and Means for IDUs to Sterilize Injection Equipment

IDUs' growing awareness of the risks of using contaminated injection equipment has increased their demand for access to sterile equipment and the means to properly sterilize it. Many current sterilization methods are ineffective. These include flushing the injection equipment with tap water between uses and heating portions of the equipment in an attempt to kill the virus (D'Aquila, Williams, 1987).

Education about sterilizing injection equipment may accompany or substitute for exchange and distribution programs. Studies demonstrate that commonly available decontaminants, including household bleach and isopropyl alcohol, are effective in killing HIV in vitro. Outreach programs usually promote the use of bleach over isopropyl alcohol; some fear that otherwise, IDUs might substitute less potent forms of alcohol (such as wine, beer, or whiskey) or ingest the isopropyl alcohol itself. Programs instruct IDUs to flush equipment three times with bleach and three times with clean, preferably sterile, water (Preston, Armsby, 1990). Others have given IDUs small vials of bleach and instructions, in written or cartoon form (Watters, 1987).

The potential public health benefits from bleach programs resemble those of distribution and exchange programs: reducing the incidence of blood-borne infections among IDUs and providing the opportunity, through contact with the bleach program, for referrals to treatment, counseling on safer sexual practices, and access to other social services. Bleach programs are less effective than exchange programs in controlling or tracking the quantity of injection equipment in a community.

Injecting drug users in San Francisco have accepted the use of bleach to decontaminate injection equipment (Stryker, Smith, 1993). Whether using bleach will achieve the goal of reducing HIV transmission among IDUs under actual conditions is unknown and is the subject of study (Vlahov, Munoz, et al., 1991). After recent review of the available scientific evidence, an expert panel concluded that although bleach disinfection of contaminated needles and syringes according to Centers for Disease Control recommendations is likely to be effective, studies have not been able to demonstrate decreased HIV infections attributable to bleach (Normand, Vlahov, et al., 1995). The failure of studies, to date, to demonstrate the efficacy of bleach programs may be due to several factors. IDUs' adherence to the six-step cleaning procedure may decrease over time or vary depending on where they shoot drugs. One limitation on efficacy in settings such as "shooting galleries" is the lack of uncontaminated water with which to flush the equipment. Moreover, recent data raise questions about the benefits of bleach cleaning. Bleach has been found to be less effective against HIV in blood than in a cell culture or cell-free state. Studies have shown that a six-second cleaning with a ten percent dilution of household bleach fails to remove clotted blood contaminated with HIV (National Institute on Drug Abuse—U.S., 1993).

Given the uncertainty of the data, the central issue from a human rights perspective is not whether governments distribute bleach packets. The important point is that governments fully educate IDUs and that individuals receive and impart information freely (UDHR, Art. 26.1, 26.2; ICESCR, Art. 13.1; UDHR, Art. 19; ICCPR, Art. 19). Injecting drug users cannot protect their health and lives without comprehensible information and the means to obtain necessary sterile equipment (see the "Right to Health" ICESCR, Art. 12[c]).

Condoms

Using condoms to prevent the exchange of bodily fluids during sexual activity substantially decreases the risk of HIV transmission. Researchers conducted a longitudinal study of 256 HIV-discordant couples over a period that ranged from twenty to twenty-four months. The study recorded a total of approximately 15,000 instances of sexual intercourse. Among the 124 couples reported using condoms during every episode of sexual intercourse), none of the HIV-negative partners seroconverted. By contrast, the estimated cumulative incidence of seroconversion among 121 couples who used condoms inconsistently was 12.7 percent after twenty-four months of follow-up (De Vincenzi, 1994). The proper use of condoms also reduces the transmission of sexually transmitted infections (STIs) and prevents pregnancies. Programs to minimize unsafe sexual practices by promoting the use of condoms may target the general public or specific groups such as gay men or adolescents. Condoms may be sold in pharmacies or other retail stores, bars, hotels, or vending machines. They may be distributed free of charge by health care workers, family planning clinics, educators, or activists. In some situations, condom distribution has been coupled with voluntary or mandatory health education or counseling to prevent STIs or pregnancy. Other efforts have focused on ensuring that condoms are widely available.

Authorities may have to overcome a variety of sociocultural, moral, religious, or legal obstacles to implement condom programs. In many places where condom use is rare, men associate them with infertility and a loss of pleasure and spontaneity (United Nations, 1990a; Elias, Heise, 1993). Some religious leaders oppose any artificial form of birth control, including condoms (Pope John Paul II, 1989). In some countries, the commercial media may block the advertising broadcast of any information related to condoms (Stryker, Samuels, et al., 1993).

Data are incomplete on how effective condom programs are in increasing consistent condom use and, therefore, in preventing HIV transmission. In part, this reflects the difficulty of measuring the isolated effect of any one prevention program. Most studies cannot track the true incidence of HIV; they must use surrogate markers such as the number of condoms distributed or sold, the behavioral changes reported, and the incidence of STIs. The effect of other AIDS prevention messages can also interfere with the evaluation of condom programs. Moreover, few data exist because few researchers have studied certain types of interventions, such as those in schools (Kirby, 1993).

In spite of these difficulties, many countries report that condom programs show encouraging results. One approach to increase condom use integrates marketing research, product conception and promotion, pricing, and physical distribution components. For instance, in Zaire, a social marketing campaign to sell condoms under the brand name "Prudence" increased condom distribution from 0.5 million to 18 million between 1987 and 1991. In Thailand, efforts to achieve 100 percent condom use by commercial sex workers markedly increased condom use and decreased STI rates. In one Thai province where reported condom use among commercial sex workers rose to nearly 100 percent, the incidence of STIs among the sex workers dropped from thirteen percent to 0.3–0.5 percent. Programs in Switzerland, Zimbabwe, Mexico, Tanzania, and Rwanda have all reported either greater distribution, sale, or use of condoms, or fewer STIs where this was measured (World Health Organization, Global Programme on AIDS, 1992g).

By contrast, social marketing efforts to promote condom use in the United States have been modest. "Historically, United States condom marketers have struggled against the notoriety of their product and its association in the public mind with extramarital sex, promiscuity, and prostitution" (DeJong, 1989). Studies in North America suggest that condom distribution programs are most effective when they are accompanied by educational messages and promotions (Kirby, Waszak, et al., 1991).

Public education programs that promote the use of condoms and candidly inform students about sex may appear to condone premarital or extramarital sexual activity. Religious or community leaders may oppose such messages because they conflict with moral values or threaten religious beliefs (UDHR, Art. 18; ICCPR, Art. 18.1, 18.2). Such instruction might also undermine parents' rights to determine their children's religious and moral education (UDHR, Art. 26.3; ICESCR, Art. 13.3; ICCPR, Art. 18.4; Commonwealth Secretariat, 1990; Stryker, Samuels, et al., 1993; see also this chapter, Prevention and Education). On the other hand, many school-based programs allow parents some control over whether their children may obtain condoms; schools may require parental permission or respect parental requests to exclude children. Some parents in the United States have removed their children on religious grounds from otherwise-mandatory AIDS education classes (*Ware v. Valley Stream High School District*, 1989).

Human rights violations may occur where government, religious, or private entities block efforts to inform and enable individuals to protect themselves from HIV infection. Government or individual attempts to censor instructional content or to prevent communities from exchanging information burden the right to information (see Chapter 1: Freedom of Opinion and Expression). The danger of censorship is that in crafting a prevention message or program that offends no one, authorities may also render it ineffective to those who need it. Messages that are tailored to specific communities and cultures both respect human rights and effectively achieve public health gains (Commonwealth Secretariat, 1990).

In some cases, providing information and the methods for self-protection may not be enough. More fundamental human rights problems may prevent people from successfully exercising the available means. Discrimination against women, particularly women with low social and economic status and little power within the family, can render the promotion and even distribution of condoms relatively ineffective in some societies. Women may have scant influence over whether condoms are used. Efforts to improve women's status generally, or, specifically, to protect their rights to property, custody of their children, and support in cases of divorce or widowhood, may be necessary additions to a comprehensive AIDS control strategy. (For more discussion of the relationship between discrimination and other human rights violations and women's vulnerability to HIV infection, see Chapter 1: Nondiscrimination; Freedom from Slavery and Similar Practices.) Alternatively, developing harm reduction strategies that women control increases their ability to protect themselves. One example is the female condom, which has been tested and is now sold in several countries (Liskin, Sakondhavat, 1992). The female condom, when properly used, provides effective protection from infection with HIV and other STIs. However, it is obvious to both partners while being used and, thus, requires the male partner's acquiescence. In contrast, women's health advocates seek development of a microbicide, which could inactivate or "kill" the virus when used before or after intercourse and which could be used surreptitiously to prevent transmission during consensual or nonconsensual sex (Elias, Heise, 1993).

Conclusion

Harm reduction strategies pose complex questions from a human rights perspective; they often involve competing claims. Policymakers must carefully and sensitively weigh the interests of parents and religious and community leaders against individuals' rights to education and the free flow of information. The WHO acknowledges the potential efficacy of harm reduction strategies. To prevent HIV transmission among IDUs, it recommends that programs include access to clean injection equipment, education about decontamination, and medical treatment to end drug dependency. The WHO also supports improved access to condoms as part of a primary prevention program (World Health Organization, 1989e, 1987g).

Sensitivity to human rights concerns is indispensable to effective harm reduction approaches. Beneficial strategies include public discussion, community members' involvement in program design and implementation, and instruction about the programs' public health value. Officials should place harm reduction strategies firmly within the context of a complete prevention program that includes education about HIV transmission, abstinence, condom use, and access to drug treatment, health care, and other social services. The likely result is a program that reflects the community's values and improves public health.

Governments have an affirmative duty to educate the community about HIV/AIDS based on individuals' rights to education, free expression, and life. To this end, governments should explore, if not provide, access to the means of individual protection even if such strategies are imperfect or objectionable to some members of the community. Thus viewed, harm reduction strategies involving condoms and sterile injection equipment are an option that might be considered by every public health authority.

RESEARCH ON HUMAN SUBJECTS: INTERNATIONAL ETHICAL GUIDELINES

Introduction

Biomedical, behavioral, and epidemiological research are critical in controlling the HIV pandemic. Large-scale trials to develop effective drugs and vaccines are underway in several parts of the world. Researchers are seeking to understand the motivation for behaviors that place individuals at risk for HIV, and how best to alter these behaviors. Epidemiologic surveillance and research are designed to track the epidemic within populations and to assist public health officials in developing well-targeted strategies to slow the spread of the virus and to provide care for persons with the disease.

The urgency to discover scientific answers to many of the questions posed by the pandemic can expose research subjects to exploitation and risk. Individuals may face not only the physical risks inherent in research but also discrimination and a loss of autonomy and privacy. Furthermore, research may profoundly affect a community's customs, morals, and pride.

Article 7 of the International Covenant on Civil and Political Rights states: "No one shall be subjected to torture or to cruel, inhuman or degrading treatment or punishment. In particular, no one shall be subjected without his free consent to medical or scientific experimentation." A series of ethical codes developed in the aftermath of World War II contain more detailed ethical guidelines on the conduct of human subject research. The Nuremberg Code of Ethics, which was issued in 1947 to protect the rights of human subjects, was one of the most important outcomes of the Nuremberg war trials. The Nuremberg Code sought to prevent a repetition of the atrocities committed by Nazi research physicians. Its first principle is that no human experimentation can occur without the subject's free and informed consent.

Since the Nuremberg Code, several international bodies have developed potent ethical guidelines for researchers. The World Medical Association adopted the Helsinki Declaration in 1964 and has now revised it three times. The Declaration has universal application in proposing the minimum standards of ethical research, including informed consent and confidentiality.

In 1982, the Council of International Organizations of Medical Sciences (CIOMS) issued Proposed Guidelines for the Conduct of Human Subject Research (World Health Organization, 1982). The document's purpose was to explain how ethical principles relate to research, particularly in developing countries. CIOMS, in conjunction with the WHO, also published the International Guidelines for Ethical Review of Epidemiologic Studies in 1991. These guidelines address the impact of large-scale research on entire populations. In 1993, in collaboration with the WHO, CIOMS revised and expanded its 1982 guidelines to reflect the growth in drug and vaccine trials, transnational research, and studies involving vulnerable populations. The International Ethical Guidelines for Biomedical Research Involving Human Subjects (Council of International Organizations of Medical Sciences, 1993) helps countries (particularly developing ones) to define national priorities on the ethics of biomedical research, to apply ethical standards in local circumstances, and to establish committees to review research involving human subjects.

International guidelines on human subject research address a wide band of ethical concerns. They seek to protect the dignity and integrity of individuals and communities, including vulnerable populations that are nondominant, poor, disenfranchised, compromised, persecuted, or restricted. This section explores five central themes in human subject research: informed consent, protection of vulnerable persons, protection of privacy, ethical review procedures, and distributive justice in international collaborative research. (For further discussion of human rights and ethical norms in AIDS-related human subject research, see Chapter 5: Case Study 2: Part B.)

Informed Consent of Subjects

Guideline 1 of CIOMS (1993) states that "for all biomedical research involving human subjects, the investigator must obtain the informed consent of the prospective subject or, in the case of an individual who is not capable of giving informed consent, the proxy consent of a properly authorized representative."

Informed consent can only be given by a competent individual who has received full and comprehensible information about the study's nature, purpose, benefits, and risks.

The person must agree to participate without undue influence. Informed consent is a central ethical requirement; it holds that mentally capable persons should control decisions regarding their health, well-being, and dignity. Ethical research always places the desires and needs of the subject over those of the investigator (Council of Europe, 1990). The requirement of informed consent helps to prevent abuse by overzealous governments or researchers who may be pressured to conduct expeditious investigations into overwhelming health problems.

As a tool to preserve human dignity and health, however, consent is increasingly being questioned. Many factors can subvert a truly informed and voluntary relationship between a clinician/researcher and patient/subject: A fine line exists between therapy and research; a lack of access to innovative treatment may prompt a subject to volunteer for a clinical trial; researchers often offer financial or other inducements for participation in a trial; researchers and human subjects often differ in linguistic and cultural understandings; and legal consent forms tend to be complex. Problems with informed consent are exacerbated in urban communities and poor rural areas where illiteracy and mistrust based on race, culture, or social class may undermine the researcher/subject relationship. In international collaborative research, the practical obstacles to obtaining consent are even more evident. They stem from marked inequities of power and resources, vast differences in laws and culture, and pressing problems of disease, hunger, illiteracy, and poverty (Ekunwe, Kessel, 1984).

International guidelines recognize that informed consent does not fully protect individuals and communities. Therefore, independent ethical review of research proposals must complement informed consent requirements.

In some communities, the very concept of respect for persons as individuals conflicts "with more relational definitions of the person found in other societies . . . which stress the embeddedness of the individual within society and define a person by his or her relations to others" (Christakis, 1988; Ajayi, 1980; Adityanjee, 1986; Levine, 1982). For example, in West Africa and the Indian subcontinent, deference may be given to clinicians, healers, and elders (Indian Council of Medical Research, 1980). Decisions are characteristically made in consultation with leaders during village meetings (Hall, 1989). If a community or family representative has given permission, the notion of an informed refusal by the individual may not even arise. In West Africa, obedience to tribal leaders powerfully influences participation in research (Henderson, Davis, et al., 1973). Where indigenous cultural beliefs exist, the research may assume a wholly different meaning than intended or understood by Northern/Western scientists (Ajayi, 1980).

Giving impoverished persons in the least developed countries money, drugs, and food to elicit consent to participate in clinical trials may obviate the element of choice (Adityanjee, 1986; Ajayi, 1980). Yet, providing reasonable compensation to impoverished subjects who may spend time away from life-sustaining work is entirely justified.

Despite the problem of imposing a Northern/Western concept of informed consent on developing countries, some culturally appropriate agreement to participate in research remains essential. "While a consent procedure must be adapted to accommodate cultural mores, there must always be a requirement for consent from the individual pro-spective subject" (World Health Organization, 1989j).

Many societies emphasize the community or family leaders' assent to research. Within the community, the leader may represent its interest as much as any individual. The community leader's consent, therefore, cannot substitute for the individual's consent, but it may constitute an additional and culturally appropriate step in obtaining permis-sion for research.

Large-scale research raises the issue of how a population might agree to participate in research. Specifically, can a legitimate community representative grant permission on behalf of the community's members? Surely, community leaders cannot truly con-sent for the entire population, for they likely would not know each individual's deci-sion. But perhaps "consent" is not the proper word; each of the traditional elements is lacking: specific information about risks and benefits, voluntariness, and competency. A better characterization may be to recommend consultations with leaders to obtain a "community consensus" on population-based research. Nonetheless, researchers have a duty to obtain individual consent as well. These concepts—individual consent, per-mission, and consensus—constitute cumulative ethical obligations to be examined in light of both international human rights norms and local cultural and ethical beliefs.

Protection for Vulnerable People and Populations

Not every person can give competent, voluntary consent to research. Some people have limited autonomy due to, for example, youth, mental illness, or cognitive impairment. Others, such as prisoners, or in some countries, military personnel, are so restricted in their freedoms and so subject to authority that their consent is not fully voluntary. For other individuals, research may be associated with heightened risks. For instance, a pregnant woman may be at higher risk because of her condition, and the fetus may be unnecessarily exposed to harm. Strict criteria must apply before persons with limited capacity, restricted freedoms, or heightened risks can participate in a clinical trial. On the other hand, routinely excluding women of child-bearing age, pregnant women, or young people from research may deprive these groups of equal benefit from scientific advances because researchers cannot conduct basic research on disease progression, drug safety, and efficacy.

Ethical principles compel a special justification for research on vulnerable popula-tions, one that seeks to protect them from exploitation and harm as well as from dis-crimination in access to the benefits of research. A vulnerable population may be de-fined as a class of individuals or groups that are nondominant, subservient, or subject to restrictions in the culture in which they live. These populations might include a minor-ity race, religion, or ethnic group; indigenous people; or aliens. These groups may retain social, cultural, economic, and political characteristics that are distinct from other seg-ments of the national population (United Nations, 1990b).

What circumstances might justify research on vulnerable groups? A particularly positive "benefit to burden" ratio may be one such circumstance. First, establishing that the health advantages clearly outweigh the risks would help to protect the subjects. Second, the problem to be studied should clearly relate to the population's health problems. A study of HIV and TB, for example, in an area where the diseases are endemic may be fully justified, despite the population's vulnerability. The principle of justice, of course, requires that the vulnerable population have access to the present and future benefits of research. Third, one must respect the population's right to self-direction and protection from harm. The voices of vulnerable populations should be heard not only on issues of subject selection but also on the ethical conduct and outcomes of the research (See the discussion of "persons with HIV infection or at risk of contracting HIV infection" in CIOMS, 1993).

Consider the ethical quandary over HIV antiviral or vaccine research in Africa or Southeast Asia, particularly if conducted with a vulnerable group such as prostitutes. Researchers may more expeditiously perform field trials in endemic areas because of the greater incidence of infection. Thus, they can obtain reliable results more quickly and less expensively than in other areas. However, due to the prohibitive cost, the local population may never see the benefit of a safe and efficacious drug or vaccine; a costly antiviral agent might be low on the host country's health care priorities. In a vaccine trial for HIV, beneficent treatment of persons would require counseling subjects to avoid high-risk behavior. This would undoubtedly result in relatively smaller measured effects, requiring a larger sample size to demonstrate the vaccine's efficacy.

Cost and expediency alone rarely suffice to ethically justify subject selection. The key questions are: How much benefit and harm might accrue to the population? Are adequate laboratory or animal models available to predict efficacy and risk? What are the reasons that other, less vulnerable, subjects cannot be used, and can they be used in parallel?

Research subjects may obtain special benefits, sometimes of considerable worth. Certain persons and populations ought not to be excluded from those benefits because of their vulnerability. To exclude these populations from participating in research may deny them their only realistic hope of effective treatment. Further, if drugs or vaccines have not been tested on, for example, African populations, women, or children, determining their effect on these populations will be difficult. Barring these groups from research impedes scientific understanding of their health needs and delays promising interventions. The inability to generalize research results to vulnerable populations may require that those populations be involved in clinical trials. A balance needs to be struck between protecting vulnerable people and providing them with the benefits of therapeutic innovation.

Protecting the Privacy of People and Populations

Research subjects possess a right to privacy on several levels: the right to space—physically, personally, and socially (e.g., absence of intrusive questioning or surveillance); a right to control disclosure of information about health, behavior, or life circumstances (e.g., drug use or sexual history); and the right to maintain intimacy and confidences in personal, family, and social relationships (e.g., interactions with sexual partners, spouses, and professional counselors).

Linking sensitive information to an individual can inflict both tangible and intangible harms. The person could face tangible harms such as discrimination by employers, educators, landlords, or insurers (Gostin, 1990a,b), or personal violation and shame. Each culture manifests its own mores about confidential information and relationships. It behooves researchers from other countries to learn about and be sensitive to local customs and religious and personal beliefs regarding the sanctity of confidential information.

From an investigator's perspective, maintaining confidentiality has utilitarian value. Recruiting and retaining human subjects is more difficult if researchers cannot ensure the confidentiality of the information obtained during the trial. Maintaining confidentiality is consistent with international documents that address research. Specifically, Guideline 12 of CIOMS (1993) states: "The investigator must establish secure safeguards of the confidentiality of research data. Subjects should be told of the limits to the investigators' ability to safeguard confidentiality and of the anticipated consequences of breaches of confidentiality."

Ethical principles of privacy and confidentiality apply to populations as well as individuals. The potential for violating privacy rights is formidable where wide-scale collection, transfer, and use of information occurs. Sharing information about a group can harm both the group and its members. Sophisticated computer technology that stores and shares personal data with countless sources only heightens the concern over privacy, stigmatization, and discrimination within populations. Information can be obtained from, and transferred to, government agencies (e.g., census, vital statistics, revenue collection, health, social services, and defense), schools, health care services, and police (Gostin, 1995b; Capron, 1989).

Data suggesting that particular groups are more likely to be infected with, and hence, capable of transmitting communicable or sexually transmitted diseases may reinforce irrational fears. Data that create or intensify negative cultural stereotypes can be particularly hurtful. Examples include research purporting to demonstrate that HIV originated in Africa (Tabor, Gerety, et al., 1990) or that homosexuals, drug abusers, and commercial sex workers intentionally spread HIV.

Ethical Review Procedures

Guideline 14 of CIOMS 1993 addresses the responsibilities of ethical review committees. "All proposals to conduct research involving human subjects must be submitted for review and approval to one or more independent ethical and scientific review committees. The investigator must obtain such approval of the proposal to conduct research before the research is begun."

Society has a dual responsibility to ensure that all drugs, devices, and vaccines under investigation in human subjects meet adequate standards of safety and that the Declaration of Helsinki is applied in all biomedical research on human subjects. Scientific and ethical review cannot be clearly separated; scientifically unsound research is itself unethical since it may expose human subjects to risk or inconvenience for no valid purpose.

Independent committees should review international collaborative research in both the sponsoring and host countries. Committees may be created at the national or local level and consist of individuals capable of adequately reviewing all significant scientific and ethical aspects of the research. Committees reviewing HIV research should consider the advantages of including as members or consultants persons who are living with HIV infection or AIDS.

Ethical review in the host and sponsoring countries is essential to conducting high-quality, ethical research. Committees in the host country tend to have a greater understanding of and sensitivity to the community's concerns, customs, and beliefs. Respecting the integrity of people and communities can foster cooperation.

Distributive Justice in International Collaborative Research

As is the international human rights community, the field of research ethics is currently debating the issue of positive and negative rights. Widespread agreement exists on the negative rights of informed consent; less consensus exists on the positive entitlements of human subjects and their communities to the benefits of research.

Consider a case in which researchers from a developed country undertake a large field trial for a vaccine or drug in a developing country. During the trial, what responsibilities, if any, do the investigators have to the subjects and to the wider community? What responsibilities, if any, do they have once the trial is over? Traditional ethical principles require that subjects be protected during the clinical trial, at least from harm arising directly from participation. This would mean that qualified clinicians carefully observe any adverse effects of the research on subjects and provide immediate treatment. Once the drug or vaccine has been shown to be efficacious, the study should cease so that those in the control group can be treated.

Furthermore, do investigators have a duty not merely to avoid directly harming subjects, but also affirmatively to protect the participants' health and well-being by providing reasonable preventive and health services? Researchers should view subjects as whole persons with diverse health needs, and not merely as tools for research purposes. The principle of distributive justice holds that a primary ethical justification for choosing to study vulnerable populations is to confer upon them benefits in exchange for participation. Benefits might include access to the drug or vaccine featured in the study design, as well as risk reduction and health care services. When persons on the margins of survival donate productive time to scientific endeavors, they ought to receive at least minimal services in return.

Seen from the subjects', rather than the researchers', perspective, the completion of the study and the withdrawal of services will likely precipitate a sense of loss and unmet expectations. Sponsors and researchers who leave behind some continuing capacity to meet subjects' needs, even if at a reduced level, help ensure cooperation regarding future research projects.

If a drug or vaccine is shown to be safe and effective, what responsibility, if any, does the research team have with respect to the local population? Persons who sponsor and conduct research in developing communities obtain a substantial benefit by gaining access to otherwise-unavailable populations. In contrast, the populations bear the risks and burdens of research. Industry may benefit financially from government subsidies to develop a product. In some countries, industry is also permitted to set the product's price at whatever level it wishes. The commercial developers of new drugs or vaccines stand to make substantial profits in the marketplace. Arguments for making the product more widely available to the local population, then, are based upon the mutual exchange of benefits and the equities of access to essential health improvements irrespective of the ability to pay. The World Health Organization Consultation on candidate HIV vaccines noted that justice requires that the "population in which the vaccine is tested is entitled to first priority in receiving the vaccine after its safety and efficacy have been established" (World Health Organization, 1989h).

Research conducted in developing countries sometimes inequitably allocates benefits and burdens. For example, all areas of the world benefit from the development of an effective vaccine or pharmaceutical, but a significant burden of the research rests on poorer developing countries. At the same time, economic poverty and underdeveloped medical services foreseeably prevent poorer countries from buying and distributing beneficial preventive or therapeutic agents (Christakis, 1989). It would be unjust if the populations that bore the most significant burdens were to reap the fewest rewards.

The idea that research subjects and their communities have an ethical entitlement to benefits after the research is concluded is controversial and is not yet fully recognized in international ethical codes. In practice, the best way to resolve this issue is through careful discussion and agreement among sponsors, researchers, and subjects. If all parties to the trial agree at the outset on the equitable distribution of burdens and benefits, miscommunication and unrealistic expectations can be lessened, if not avoided.

Commentators have questioned the overall mix of types of research conducted in developing countries, as well as investigators' duties to ensure that the research leads to appropriate public health or treatment interventions (DeCock, Ekpini, et al., 1994). In the first decade of the epidemic, the majority of the 559 AIDS-related research studies that were conducted in Africa, and reviewed by WHO staff, concerned descriptive epidemiology, perinatal transmission of HIV, and assessment of knowledge, attitudes, and practice (Heymann, Bres, et al., 1990). Little research was aimed at developing the best clinical interventions for persons with HIV infection or at managing HIV in a resource poor environment. Although the study concerned only research in Africa, research in other areas of the developing world may exhibit a similar mix of studies. Ethical and human rights standards—as well as practical considerations—suggest that the international community should adjust the mix of research conducted in developing countries to address more closely the needs of both developing and industrialized nations.

Research on AIDS and HIV in Africa has produced important information for other countries and regions in their fight against AIDS. Human subjects who bear a disproportionate burden of research should be entitled to share in the benefits. Likewise, the populations that provide researchers with invaluable data about HIV, its mode of transmission, and its impact on societies are also entitled to benefits that meet their particular needs. In the case of Africa, Heymann and colleagues outline a number of areas where necessary research would produce a substantial public health benefit, including evaluating various HIV prevention and education strategies, especially those aimed at youth; measuring the impact of HIV testing on prevention programs; developing new approaches to HIV surveillance; improving tuberculosis control; integrating sexually transmitted disease control into primary care; implementing more effective blood donor deferral systems; reducing the unnecessary use of blood and blood products; and empowering women to enable them to avoid HIV infection (1990).

International human rights norms recognize the right of all persons to share in the benefits of scientific progress and its applications (UDHR, Art. 27; ICESCR, Art. 15; see also Chapter 1: The Right to Share the Benefits of Scientific and Technological Progress). This provision aims to bring essential scientific advances to not only those who can pay for them, or who participated in their development, but to everyone who might benefit from them. Under international human rights standards, investigators may be obligated to balance the types of research that they conduct in the developing world and to address the research population's specific health needs, which may differ from those of industrialized countries.

Finally, governments which have up to now cooperated in the design and execution of studies driven mostly by Western scientists' research needs, in the future may be less eager to collaborate unless research projects also address their countries' particular needs. Foremost among their concerns is likely to be practical solutions for caring for ever-growing numbers of persons with HIV infection in environments that have minimal resources (DeCock, Ekpini, et al., 1994).

5

Case Studies Raising Critical Questions in HIV Policy and Research: Balancing Public Health Benefits and Human Rights Burdens

In this final chapter, we present three case studies that raise critical questions regarding HIV policy and research. Using the Human Rights Impact Assessment outlined in Chapter 3, we balance the public health benefits and human rights burdens. Because the exercise is intended to challenge the reader with some of the complex policy and research questions facing policymakers, scientists, and public health professionals, we intentionally avoid arriving at a "correct" answer. The Human Rights Impact Assessment tool is applied to (1) sort and distill the issues; (2) clarify whether the policy would achieve a valid public health objective; (3) identify the potential risks, detriments, and impacts on human rights; and (4) guide the search for less restrictive, more effective, alternatives.

The cases involve discrimination and the transmission of HIV and tuberculosis in an occupational health care setting, breast-feeding in the least developed countries, and confidentiality and the right of sexual partners to know of potential exposure to HIV.

Public policymakers using the Human Rights Impact Assessment will review primarily health officials' authorization and use of state power to protect and promote health. Those designing or implementing health interventions at the national, provincial, or city level have the greatest scope of authority and discretion in creating or modifying policy. However, even health care administrators and providers in individual institutions can use this assessment to guide their policy decisions, although their discretion may be bound by other legal and nonlegal constraints. The case studies include examples of policies designed and implemented by both public health officials and private institutions.

CASE STUDY 1: A HEALTH CARE WORKER WITH HIV INFECTION

In areas with a high prevalence of *Mycobacterium tuberculosis* (TB), mounting evidence indicates that transmission occurs in hospitals, affecting both patients and health care workers.[1] In places such as New York City, a growing concern is the spread of multidrug resistant tuberculosis (MDR-TB) in hospital settings.

A nurse in the emergency department of a city hospital operated by the public health department performs preliminary physical exams, takes patient histories, starts IVs, gives injections, cleans wounds, and prepares patients for admission or transport. He occasionally assists with emergency births, controls combative patients, and performs cardiopulmonary resuscitation.

Experiencing some vague physical symptoms, the nurse visits his physician at the hospital where the nurse works. After discussing with his physician the risks and benefits of HIV-antibody testing, the nurse consents to testing. Although the nurse is asymptomatic, the test results confirm that he has HIV infection. The physician is concerned that the nurse is at risk of contracting TB on the job and may transmit HIV or TB infection to patients. Without the nurse's knowledge or permission, the physician informs the nurse's supervisor of the diagnosis. The supervisor informs the hospital administration. Immediately thereafter, the administration promulgates a policy "to protect health care workers and patients" and transfers the nurse from the emergency department to a nonpatient-contact position at the same pay. The new position does not afford the same opportunities for acquiring skills or promotion as the nurse's previous position. The nurse, displeased by the transfer, requests a return to direct patient care.

Based on the Human Rights Impact Assessment, should the hospital maintain or modify its new policy?

Assessment

Is the hospital justified in either (1) protecting the nurse from contracting TB from patients or (2) protecting patients from contracting HIV or TB from the nurse?

Analyze the Facts

The first step in evaluating a policy that may burden human rights is a thorough and objective analysis of the facts. Authorities should gather broad-based information; that is, they should avoid relying on single sources of information and should scrutinize a

---

1. This case is based on background information on tuberculosis in New York (Garrett, Woodward 1992). The situation described here is purely fictional (see also Gostin, 1995).

data for possible biases. Persons other than hospital administrators or physicians (e.g., infectious disease experts, environmental engineers, industrial hygienists, public health officials, union representatives, and persons with HIV infection) can serve as valuable resources.

Health care workers in urban centers face an increasing risk of occupational exposure to TB. The risk is greatest in places that serve populations at risk of infection. In the city where the nurse works, these populations include members of certain racial and ethnic minority groups, recent immigrants from countries with high rates of TB, current and past prison inmates, injecting drug users (IDUs), and homeless people. Health care professionals who work in emergency departments, outpatient or drug treatment clinics, or settings where patients are induced to cough for diagnostic or therapeutic reasons are at a heightened risk of occupational exposure to TB (Centers for Disease Control and Prevention, 1994b).

In some settings, these risks have produced significant rates of occupational infection. Over the past eighteen months at another local hospital, one-half of the medical staff reportedly became infected with TB. Twelve staff members developed active disease, and five, who were HIV positive, died of TB (Garrett, Woodward, 1992).

Public health officials are troubled about the upsurge in MDR-TB cases. Studies of more than 500 TB cases in two large teaching hospitals revealed no cases of drug-resistant TB between 1987 and mid-1989. From mid-1989 through early 1991, however, nineteen hospital workers contracted MDR-TB; six of them died. Forty patients contracted MDR-TB as hospital in-patients; twenty-six of them died by the end of 1991 (Garrett, Woodward, 1992). During the same period, at least 100 city residents were diagnosed with MDR-TB; six died.

Persons with HIV or other immunocompromising conditions are more susceptible to TB infection and substantially more likely to develop active disease than persons with normal immune systems. Only ten percent of nonimmunocompromised persons who are infected with TB ever develop active disease. In contrast, HIV-positive persons who are infected with TB have an eight to ten percent chance per year of developing active disease (Selwyn, Hartel, et al., 1989). The majority of persons infected with both HIV and TB will eventually develop active TB if untreated.

Furthermore, persons dually infected with HIV and MDR-TB are likely to die within a short period of time. Seventy to ninety percent of these patients die from TB, one-half within four to sixteen weeks (Snider, Roper, 1992).

The conditions that precipitate transmission of TB in hospitals are not unique to a particular facility or locale. The factors include a shortage of properly ventilated isolation rooms, the difficulty of implementing effective infection control measures where undiagnosed TB patients are present (e.g., emergency departments, outpatient clinics, medical and pediatric units), laboratory delays in diagnosing TB and identifying drug resistance, and staff unfamiliarity with the signs and symptoms of TB (Centers for Disease Control and Prevention, 1994b). Moreover, the high cost of many necessary measures impedes infection control efforts (Gostin, 1995). The cost of improving municipal hospitals in a single large city in the United States is estimated to be in the millions (U.S. dollars).

If the nurse is not already infected, evidence of the recent TB outbreak infecting one-half of a nearby hospital's emergency room staff strongly suggests that he is at risk of occupational infection. Studies indicate that exposure to TB is most likely to occur in emergency departments and waiting areas for undiagnosed patients. The increasing incidence of MDR-TB in the city suggests that both health care workers and patients are at risk of contracting this pernicious and recalcitrant form of TB.

We do not know whether the nurse is currently infected with TB. Like all health care workers, he should be screened periodically for TB infection and disease and offered appropriate prophylaxis or treatment (Centers for Disease Control and Prevention, 1995f, 1994b). Screening an HIV-positive person for TB somewhat complicates the skin test (PPD—purified protein derivative of tuberculin); the test may produce false results in immunosuppressed persons. Providers who test the nurse should modify their procedures to detect TB more accurately in this situation.

The environment of the emergency department presents several characteristics conducive to TB transmission. Persons with undiagnosed but active TB or reactivated TB frequent the emergency room, often for extended periods of time. On average, a TB patient in this city waits twenty hours before being either treated or admitted (Arno, Murray, et al., 1993). The emergency department waiting area is crowded and poorly ventilated. The ventilation system recirculates rather than exhausts the air, which efficiently distributes TB-infected air droplets to all areas within the department and, perhaps, within the hospital.

The hospital should consider whether the ventilation system aerates other parts of the facility with TB-contaminated air; whether appropriate isolation rooms are available for patients diagnosed with TB; and whether the staff is alert to signs and symptoms of TB—to facilitate early diagnosis, prompt isolation, and effective treatment (Centers for Disease Control and Prevention, 1990a, 1995f).

Research suggests that the risk of HIV transmission from health care workers to patients is remote. Although HIV-positive health care workers can pose a risk of infection to patients under certain circumstances, that risk is exceedingly low. In only one instance (a dental practice) has HIV transmission from a health care worker to patients (six) been reported. A study of approximately 20,000 patients treated by fifty-seven HIV-positive health care providers found no cases of transmission from providers to patients (Centers for Disease Control and Prevention, 1993). Moreover, rigorous infection control practices, termed "universal precautions," reduce the already low risk. Despite consistent application of such measures, however, some risk remains during invasive procedures—sometimes called "exposure-prone invasive procedures"—whereby health care workers may be injured by sharp instruments and bleed on or into the patient. Examples include certain surgical and obstetrical procedures and treatment of severe trauma. The hospital should assess the nurse's responsibilities and determine whether and how often he performs exposure-prone invasive procedures while in the emergency department. The hospital should also identify the duties the nurse would perform for patients in other areas of the hospital (Centers for Disease Control and Prevention, 1991a; see also Chapter 4: The Health Care System).

The modes of transmission of TB and HIV differ in ways that substantially alter the risks from infected patients or workers. Furthermore, the risk of the nurse transmitting TB to patients differs from his risk of transmitting HIV. Tuberculosis is an airborne disease that can be transmitted through prolonged contact with patients. Unless the nurse develops active infectious tuberculosis, he poses little or no risk of transmitting the disease. The hospital might carefully monitor the nurse and remove him from patient care if he develops a sign of active disease.

Examine the Public Health Interest

The hospital should explicitly and narrowly define its policy's public health purpose. This will guide administrators' practices and facilitate an objective analysis. Here, the hospital offers two justifications for its policy: preventing health care workers with HIV infection from contracting TB and preventing transmission of HIV and TB from health care workers to patients.

The hospital has a valid public health purpose in protecting all health care workers from TB infection. Hospital administrators are responsible for implementing effective TB control measures such as risk assessment; early identification, isolation, and complete treatment of patients with infectious TB; proper engineering controls; appropriate respiratory protection programs; and education, counseling, screening, and evaluation for health care workers (Centers for Disease Control and Prevention, 1995f). Given the rates of TB infection in city hospitals, administrators and public health officials have good cause to be concerned about potential infection. Health care workers with HIV infection are particularly vulnerable to contracting TB, developing active disease, transmitting it to others, and dying from it. Preventing TB infection among HIV-infected health care workers can avert illness and death. The occurrence of MDR-TB in this city and the poor prognosis of persons who have both HIV and MDR-TB make the objective particularly compelling.

The hospital also propounds a valid public health purpose in preventing transmission of HIV and MDR-TB to patients. Hospitals have a special duty to safeguard patients' health. The hospital must initiate all reasonable precautions to protect patients from acquiring nosocomial infections.

Examine the Overall Effectiveness of the Policy

Hospital officials must demonstrate that their decision to remove the nurse from patient contact constitutes an appropriate means to achieve their goals. Specifically, the hospital must show that the policy is reasonably likely to prevent the nurse from either contracting TB within the hospital or from transmitting HIV or TB to patients. Removing the nurse from contact with patients who have active TB—and from settings like the emergency room—could significantly reduce the nurse's risk of contracting and transmitting TB to patients. Moreover, transferring the nurse essentially eliminates the already remote risk that he will transmit HIV to patients.

The reassignment policy, however, is not entirely effective, and it entails costs. Transfer will not protect from TB those health care workers with undiagnosed HIV infection, nor those who choose to not report their diagnosis to the hospital. Furthermore, the benefits of reassignment may be abrogated by lax infection control measures for HIV and TB and by the hospital's ventilation system. A ventilation system that circulates TB throughout the facility increases the risk of infection to the entire staff and all the patients. An inadequate supply of disposable needles, gloves, and protective clothing, or the failure to use universal precautions, increases the risk of HIV transmission to patients and staff. If the nurse is already infected with TB, he is at risk of developing active disease until diagnosed and fully treated; simply reassigning him will not reduce this risk.

On the other hand, eliminating all possibility of HIV transmission from health care worker to patient may not be consistent with the hospital's priorities. The hospital may achieve its goal of protecting patients from infection by an HIV-infected health care provider through the use of universal precautions (Centers for Disease Control and Prevention, 1991a). Further limiting a low risk may not be a compelling justification to seriously burden human rights or to incur substantial opportunity costs.

Examine the Issue of Consent

Informed consent is critical in public health work, not as an inert legal requirement, but as a dynamic process to enlist the understanding and cooperation of individuals in ongoing public health efforts. Here, consent is relevant to the nurse's HIV-antibody testing, his test result's disclosure, and his transfer to non–patient-care duties. Testing for HIV should occur only after the individual grants fully informed consent (see Chapter 4: Epidemiological Surveillance and Disease Control). Providers should not disclose the results without the patient's consent unless necessary to avert a serious harm to an identifiable individual (see Chapter 1: Privacy, and below, Determine the Impact on Human Rights). Here, the nurse consented to testing, but was not informed of—and did not consent to—the result's disclosure to his employer. Therefore, his consent to testing was not truly "informed" because he was denied a crucial piece of information.

The hospital did not consult with the nurse regarding reassignment. Not only did the nurse not consent to the transfer, he requests a return to his previous duties. Had the hospital administration expressed concern about the nurse's risk of infection to himself or others, perhaps he would have agreed to a transfer or other protective action. The hospital must demonstrate a compelling public health justification for its coercive intervention.

Weigh the Opportunity Costs

Implementing this policy entails certain costs and may produce unintended results. By removing the nurse from patient care, the hospital loses an experienced professional who has served in a difficult setting, the emergency department. The hospital likely can compensate for the staffing loss of one employee through training or replacement. If the hospital, however, transfers more HIV-positive health care workers to non–patient-care duties, it risks reducing its pool of skilled personnel, which may undermine its ability to provide quality care. In addition, the policy adversely affects individual workers by depriving them of their chosen work and limiting their professional opportunities.

By relying on staff transfers instead of implementing system-wide changes to prevent TB, the hospital may fail to provide a safe working environment for all its employees. Continuously exposing staff to TB could increase illness, harm morale, and induce resignations of persons who seek safer working conditions. Many urban hospitals already have difficulty fully staffing their emergency departments. The policy could exacerbate the problem.

Furthermore, by reassigning HIV-positive health care workers to non–patient-care activities, the hospital may devote less attention to and tolerate less rigorous compliance with infection control measures. This in turn could increase the risk of HIV transmission from health care workers to patients.

The hospital administration should weigh these costs against those of alternative policies. For instance, by installing or improving the ventilation system (which would benefit all workers and patients by reducing the risk of TB transmission), by providing protective equipment, and by training staff in infection-control measures, the hospital could reduce the risk of TB transmission. Moreover, by carefully monitoring the nurse's practices and adherence to universal precautions, or by modifying his activities to avoid invasive procedures, the hospital could nearly eliminate the risk of HIV transmission (see below, Search for a Range of Less Restrictive Alternatives).

Evaluate Whether the Policy Is Well-Targeted

Ideally, hospital officials will implement policies that affect as few persons as necessity requires without needlessly interfering with the rights of others. Furthermore, the hospital should avoid actions that may discriminate against already-disfavored groups.

The policy under review targets workers who are at increased risk of TB infection, but it fails to reach all those at risk. To effectively prevent TB among health care personnel with HIV, the hospital would have to reassign or otherwise protect all of them.

Therefore, the reassignment policy is underinclusive; the hospital likely employs other health care workers who, unbeknownst to it, are HIV positive. Limited to known cases of HIV infection, the policy arbitrarily singles out some employees for reassignment. Any administration attempts to identify all health care workers who have HIV, however, would be problematic; they would likely rely on invidious stereotypes, substantially invade privacy, or both. This approach could further stigmatize homosexuals, minorities, or others considered "at risk" of HIV infection. Furthermore, such an attempt might lead staff members to conceal signs of illness, impede their honest disclosure to health care providers, or discourage seeking medical treatment.

The policy is not well targeted to prevent HIV transmission. Many patient care activities do not pose even a remote risk of transmitting HIV to patients. Thus, the policy is overinclusive, or broader than necessary, to prevent HIV transmission. To avoid overbreadth, the policy should emphasize universal precautions and should apply only to HIV-positive health care workers who perform invasive procedures or activities that are most likely to expose patients to HIV.

Determine the Impact on Human Rights

The hospital must balance the efficacy of the policy against its potential human rights burdens. In doing so, it should consider the nature of the rights burdened, the invasiveness of the policy, the frequency and scope of the infringements, and their duration.

Privacy and confidentiality

The physician's disclosure of the nurse's test result without consent is troubling—from both a human rights and a public health perspective. The nurse possesses a powerful interest in protecting the confidentiality of intimate medical information (UDHR, Art. 12; ICCPR, Art. 17). Absent consent, disclosure is justified only to avoid immediate and compelling harm. Although the nurse's HIV status increases his risk of TB infection, protection of the nurse himself from possible harm is a tenuous justification for divulging highly sensitive information. The nurse's potential for transmitting HIV infection to patients constitutes an even weaker argument; no evidence exists that the nurse poses an immediate and substantial danger to others. The risk of HIV transmission from health care worker to patient is so low that it rarely, if ever, justifies disclosure to protect patients. Moreover, disclosure harms the worker professionally and perhaps personally. Here, the nurse's reassignment may alert fellow employees, family, and the community to his HIV status, which constitutes a serious breach of privacy.

Autonomy and safe working conditions

International human rights law obliges employers to protect workers from injury or illness in the workplace (ICESCR, Art. 6, 7, 12; UDHR, Art. 23; see also the Convention on Elimination of All Forms of Discrimination Against Women, Art. 11; Widdows, 1993). Accordingly, hospitals have a duty to protect health care workers from occupational exposure to infectious diseases including HIV, TB, and hepatitis B virus (HBV). Ensuring a safe working environment for health care personnel necessitates holding comprehensive infection control training programs, supplying adequate materials or equipment to prevent accidental needlesticks or airborne transmission, and providing proper ventilation and lighting. Hospitals that create a safe environment may not need to test or transfer workers to other settings.

Issues of autonomy arise when, despite all reasonable efforts, a hospital environment remains unsafe for particular personnel. Workers with HIV infection have a significant risk of contracting TB if exposed. In this case, the hospital is compelling the nurse to move to a less dangerous setting. Depriving persons of autonomy for their own good, however, is paternalistic. The nurse might argue that he alone should decide whether to assume the risk. In contrast, if the nurse poses a significant risk to others, the hospital may have the power or the duty to act.

Discrimination

Employers or other authorities should not invoke "protection" of workers or patients to mask discrimination based on invidious stereotypes or scientifically unfounded fears. Requiring differential treatment based on a worker's HIV status rather than behavior or activity is suspect, unless justified by a compelling public health reason. The hospital policy causes the nurse economic and professional hardship not experienced by his fellow workers. Reassignment is not necessary to protect patients from HIV. If the worker poses a significant risk of transmitting TB, the hospital should assign him to a position that causes as little hardship as possible.

Education and free exchange of information

Hospitals, other institutions, and the government have an obligation to educate workers and to protect and promote the free exchange of information (UDHR, Art. 19, 26; ICESCR, Art. 13; ICCPR, Art. 19). The hospital's policy fails to educate or counsel health care workers with HIV about their increased risk of contracting TB or about precautions to avoid transmitting HIV or TB to patients or partners. Moreover, the policy may limit the free exchange of information. Health care workers who fear revealing their HIV status due to professional ramifications may be reluctant to seek counseling or advice about universal precautions or behavioral changes.

Sharing the benefits of scientific advances

Health care workers have the right to share in scientific advancement and benefits (UDHR, Art. 27; ICESCR, Art. 15; Vienna Declaration and Programme of Action, 1993). By relying solely on reassignment, the hospital policy deprives infected health care workers as well as patients of the benefits of the latest TB- and HIV-prevention technology. Improved ventilation systems, ultraviolet lighting, effective isolation rooms, and personal protective devices may greatly reduce health care workers' risk of contracting TB. Appropriate supplies and education regarding universal precautions and modified practice patterns can almost eliminate the risk of HIV transmission.

The duration of these human rights burdens is substantial. The average person with HIV infection may not experience symptoms for ten years or more (Pantaleo, Graziosi, et al., 1993). Since the hospital's policy is based on the nurse's HIV status, a transfer would probably be permanent. Alternatively, the installation of a new ventilation system or other measure could abrogate the need for reassignment.

The hospital policy may increasingly burden human rights in scope and frequency. If the hospital applies the policy to all health care workers known to have HIV, infringements on basic rights will continue to increase.

Search for a Range of Less Restrictive Alternatives

A policy that effectively achieves a compelling public health objective may sometimes justify limiting human rights. A critical step in evaluating a policy is to determine whether alternate policies accomplish the same public health objective *and* impose less human rights burdens. The principle of the least restrictive alternative recommends adoption of the least intrusive but equally effective policy.

Several other measures might lower the risk of HIV-infected health care workers from contracting TB. These include eliminating the worker's contact with patients who may have TB, reassigning him to an area where patients do not have TB, improving ventilation, and providing protective clothing. City hospitals which have imposed environmental measures including improved ventilation, ultraviolet lighting, and effective isolation rooms and protective equipment combined with increased clinical awareness of the need to properly diagnose, isolate, and treat patients with cases of active TB have reduced their rates of hospital transmission of TB by up to seventy percent (Frieden, Fujiwara, et al., 1995).

The hospital has a number of options to minimize the risk of HIV-positive health care providers from transmitting HIV to patients. The hospital could allow these workers to continue to provide patient care but train them in infection control procedures and monitor their compliance. Only if the worker performs invasive procedures will a small risk of transmission remain. Training may be a preferred option where the hospital cannot afford to reassign or modify the practices of infected workers because skilled workers are not available to replace them. Alternatively, the hospital could curtail the health care worker's performance of exposure-prone or other invasive procedures and carefully monitor the worker's compliance with infection control measures. This would virtually eliminate the risk of patient infection and impose a lesser burden on the worker's rights.

Of course, alternative policies may also raise human rights concerns. Publicity about the possible transmission of HIV from health care providers to patients has led some patients and legislators to assert a "right to know" the serostatus of health care providers. The media, public, or advocacy groups may pressure institutions such as hospitals, medical associations, or governments to implement restrictive measures that needlessly burden human rights. In these situations, the least restrictive alternative principle can guide institutions and policymakers to resist such pressure and to choose less burdensome options.

Determine Whether the Policy Meets the Significant Risk Standard and Provides Fair Procedures

The hospital could conclude that removing an HIV-infected health care worker from patient care is not justified to prevent HIV infection of patients but is necessary to protect the worker from exposure to and transmission of TB to patients. After evaluating the options, the hospital might conclude that reassignment is the most effective, least restrictive alternative.

Before deciding to implement the policy, however, the hospital should make an individual determination of significant risk. This is a public health inquiry. The significant risk standard is based on a case-by-case determination of the public health risk posed to and by persons in particular circumstances. The standard will support coercive measures that burden human rights only to avert significant risks of substantial harm to others' health or safety. The standard of significant risk provides a scientifically valid basis for decisions that might otherwise be based on irrational fears, speculation, or invidious stereotypes. In this case, the hospital should determine whether the nurse's duty in the emergency department creates a significant risk that he will contract TB or will transmit TB or HIV to patients.

To determine whether the worker is at significant risk of TB infection, the hospital should consider the nature of the risk, the likely modes of transmission, the duration of the risk, the probability of transmission, and the seriousness of the harm. TB infection is potentially serious; TB can be fatal, particularly for persons who are infected with HIV or who contract MDR-TB. Emergency department work exposes the nurse to well-documented modes of TB transmission (e.g., sharing a closed space with persons who have active disease for prolonged periods of time; maintaining close contact with people who cough). The risk of exposure in the emergency department is ongoing and probably cannot be completely eliminated even with improved ventilation, lighting, and isolation facilities. The probability of infection is real and substantial, as evidenced by the staff's infection rate at a neighboring hospital. Considering the facts, the hospital could conclude that the nurse's current placement in the emergency department poses a significant risk and might transfer him to another setting. The hospital should also analyze the nurse's risk in other areas of the hospital. The hospital might conclude that the risk of TB infection is not significant if the nurse works somewhere other than the emergency or clinical outpatient departments and is not assigned to work with patients who have been diagnosed with TB.

Compared to TB, an analysis of the risk of HIV transmission from health care workers to patients reveals some important differences. Current medical knowledge holds that HIV infection produces a fatal illness and that the potential for transmission persists as long as the infected person is alive. Nonetheless, the health care worker with HIV infection does not pose a significant risk to patients because HIV is not transmitted by routine or casual contact. Communicability requires an appropriate mode of transmission. Routine contact between patients and providers in a hospital setting does not expose patients to the primary routes of HIV transmission. Most daily contact between patients and health care providers poses virtually no risk of infection to patients. Invasive procedures such as injections, drawing blood, and starting IVs pose a remote risk that can be mitigated or eliminated by universal precautions (Centers for Disease Control and Prevention, 1991a). The only activities during which HIV-positive health care workers might pose an elevated risk of exposure to patients are invasive procedures, where an injury to an HIV-positive health worker may result in an exchange of blood with the patient. The probability of this harm, although small, may justify restricting or modifying an HIV-infected health care worker's duties for these types of procedures. Given the remote probability of HIV transmission for the procedures performed by the emergency department nurse, the hospital should conclude that the significant risk test is not met here.

Where a significant risk justifies a restrictive or coercive measure, international human rights law and the concepts of natural justice or due process require authorities to provide appropriate procedural safeguards. Although the nurse is not being deprived of his liberty through isolation or comparable measures, his removal from patient care imposes substantial personal and professional burdens. Appropriate safeguards might include an examination by an independent authority of the rationale for the restrictions, affording an opportunity to challenge the facts on which the hospital bases its restrictions, and periodic policy review.

CASE STUDY 2: BREAST-FEEDING AND VERTICAL TRANSMISSION OF HIV: ASSESSMENT OF POLICY AND RESEARCH

A Policy of Artificial Feeding for an Entire or Select Population[2]

A recent seroprevalence study in a small developing country reveals a twenty-eight percent HIV prevalence rate in women attending antenatal clinics. One in every ten

2. The idea for this case study arose during a workshop on Ethical Considerations in International Research on HIV Transmission Through Breast-feeding, National Institutes of Health (U.S.), Rockville, Maryland, June 24, 1993. Dr. Angus Nicoll, MRCP (Pediatrics), Consultant Epidemiologist, HIV and STD Division, Public Health Laboratory Service, London, deserves special gratitude and recognition for her submission to the HIV workshop (Nicoll, 1993).

infants is born with HIV. In this country, the majority of women breast-feed their infants and virtually all poor women do so.

The Ministry of Health has, until now, followed the World Health Organization and United Nations International Children's Educational Fund's (WHO/UNICEF) (1992) recommendation: In areas with high infant mortality associated with infectious diseases or malnutrition, all women—including those known to be infected with HIV—should breast-feed their infants. In light of the country's high incidence of vertical transmission, however, the Ministry of Health is reevaluating its policy. The Ministry is aware of data demonstrating seroconversion of some infants due to breast-feeding (Ziegler, Cooper, et al., 1985; Palasanthiran, Ziegler, et al., 1993). Health officials know that in more affluent settings (with low infant mortality), the WHO/UNICEF recommends that HIV-infected women not breast-feed their infants. The Ministry has also learned that in many industrialized countries health officials recommend that HIV-infected mothers not breast-feed their infants.

The Ministry is considering recommending that mothers use artificial feeding (e.g., bottle-feeding, or cup and spoon feeding). Specifically, the Ministry is weighing whether to apply the recommendation to the whole population, to mothers thought to be at greater risk of HIV, or to those known to be infected. The latter option would include a program termed "voluntary confidential screening" whereby health care workers would routinely screen all women receiving care at pre- or postnatal clinics. The women would be informed of the program and tested for HIV unless they expressly refused. The results would be kept confidential. The women who test positive would be asked to attend a government health clinic for twelve to eighteen months after giving birth to monitor the health of their babies.

Assessment

Public health officials in developing countries strongly promote breast-feeding, regardless of a mother's HIV status. Public health officials reason that, overall, breast-feeding will lower infant mortality. Inadequate access to safe water and exposure to poor sanitary conditions increase the risk that bottle-fed infants will die of diarrheal disease. Furthermore, bottle-feeding poses a risk of infant malnutrition (Macedo, 1988). Breast-feeding offers two additional advantages: It supplies the infant some immunity against infection and reduces the mother's fertility.

How should the Ministry of Health evaluate the proposed policy? What human rights concerns arise?

Analyze the facts

The World Health Organization (1993) has drawn attention to breast-feeding/breast milk as a route of HIV transmission. Increasing evidence suggests that HIV may be transmitted postpartally through breast milk. Vertical transmission has been noted among women known to be infected prior to giving birth (prevalent cases) and among those who became infected while nursing (incident cases) (Van de Perre, Lepage, et al., 1992). Transmission via breast-feeding is thought to occur during the first three months after birth (Van de Perre, Simonon, et al., 1993).

A meta-analysis of epidemiological evidence has found that breast-feeding increases the risk of HIV transmission by fourteen percent for prevalent cases and by twenty-nine percent for incident cases (Dunn, Newell, et al., 1992). Although these findings have been criticized, a consensus of the scientific community believes that breast-feeding poses a risk of HIV transmission (Halsey, Boulos, et al., 1990; European Collaborative Study, 1992; Ruff, Halsey, et al., 1992; Hu, Heyward, et al., 1992). The precise level of risk, however, has yet to be determined.

Examine the public health interest

The Ministry of Health has a public health interest in preventing the vertical transmission of HIV and in protecting infants from other preventable causes of morbidity and mortality (e.g., diarrheal disease). The strength of the interest in preventing vertical transmission of HIV depends on the number of infections attributable to breast milk. In a developing country with many HIV-infected mothers, however, even a small increase in the risk of vertical transmission through breast-feeding can affect many infants. For example, assume that the maternal–infant transmission rate for breast-fed infants is thirty percent and that of bottle-fed infants is twenty-five percent. If one million children annually are breast fed by HIV-infected women, 50,000 additional children could be infected yearly (Ruff, Halsey, et al., 1992).

Examine the overall effectiveness of the policy

The Human Rights Impact Assessment recognizes that even if the public health objectives are valid, the policy may not effectively achieve them. The underlying goal of any public health program designed to benefit women and children is to reduce overall illness and death. Whether the Ministry will meet this goal depends upon the policy's public health impact. Through the strenuous and sustained efforts of national and international public health organizations, breast-feeding has substantially contributed to reducing child and maternal mortality in developing countries. A decision to recommend artificial feeding would constitute a profound reversal of policy in many developing countries. If the Ministries of Health in the least developed countries (e.g., sub-Saharan Africa) recommend artificial feeding for their entire populations, a higher net infant mortality might result (Heymann, 1990; Nicoll, Killewo, et al., 1990; Lederman, 1992). Countries with high child mortality may lose more infants to infectious and diarrheal diseases than they would save by reducing vertical transmission of HIV. The outcome, however, may be less clear in countries with intermediate child mortality (e.g., Southeast Asia or South America) where the risk of bottle-feeding is lower.

A selective policy may be more difficult to analyze. Under this approach, the Ministry would recommend bottle-feeding only for mothers known to be infected or considered to be at significant risk of HIV. Such a policy might be better targeted than the first approach because it potentially limits the number of women in the population who would forego breast-feeding. A risk exists, however, that the policy will have a spillover effect: that is, greater numbers of women—irrespective of their HIV or risk-status—will begin to bottle-feed. In the least developed countries, this unintended consequence would likely increase infant mortality associated with bottle-feeding.

Even if bottle-feeding were recommended, it may not be feasible for a significant number of women in the population because of concerns about hygiene and infant nutrition. Infant formula is expensive and its proper preparation requires, in addition to clean water, an understanding of and attention to proportions. Where resources or supplies of formula are scarce, mothers may be forced to excessively dilute the formula, leading to malnourishment. Problems posed by lack of education, infrastructure, and resources (e.g., clean water and adequate formula) would be considerable.

Examine the issue of consent

Certainly, women cannot be forced to breast- or bottle-feed. Nevertheless, the Ministry's recommendations will likely, and significantly, affect women's choices. To maximize the right of self-determination, women must be given full and accurate information about the risks and benefits of breast- and artificial feeding and counseled in a nondirective fashion which leaves them free to decide.

If the policy involves routine screening, the issue of consent becomes more pressing. Although the proposed policy would respect a woman's right to refuse testing, it does not include a timely informed consent. Informed consent to HIV testing requires full information about the nature and purpose of the testing and assent *before* the test is conducted. Informed consent should be viewed as part of a process of counseling, meaningful discussion, and permission.

Weigh the opportunity costs

For the Ministry's recommendation to have any effect on the decision to breast-feed, women must be given adequate access to safe water, affordable formula, and effective education. These measures would divert scarce resources from other public health programs (e.g., health education to reduce the number of HIV infections in women). The best opportunity for lowering the rate of pediatric HIV is to reduce HIV infections among women of child-bearing age.

The Ministry's proposed policy might carry additional costs if it inadvertently dissuades all women from breast-feeding. Consequently, non–HIV-infected women might unnecessarily consume scarce resources such as clean water and affordable formula.

A policy that involves screening pregnant women for HIV would be resource intensive. Screening would divert funding away from potentially more effective public health policies.

Evaluate whether the policy is well-targeted

A recommendation that all women bottle-feed their babies is not well targeted because it would involve women who are not infected with HIV. Under this policy, noninfected women would be advised to alter behaviors that are healthiest for them and their infants. A policy focused only on HIV-positive women would more accurately reach infants at risk of contracting HIV from nursing.

Determine the impact on human rights

A policy that simply offers health information and guidance to women without screening, at face value, minimally burdens human rights. No apparent coercion, loss of privacy, or discrimination exists. When examined more closely, however, the policy harbors the potential to significantly burden human rights.

The United Nations Declaration on Human Rights established a right to health and to life. The Declaration imposes special protections for children. The United Nations Declaration of the Rights of the Child (1959) specifies that states have a particular obligation to ensure that children grow and develop in a healthy and normal manner. This includes the right to nutrition and medical services.

A government that urges women to forgo traditional cultural breast-feeding practices retains a special obligation to ensure that mothers and infants can thrive with artificial feeding. Moreover, the policy may have irreversible consequences; once a woman has begun to bottle-feed, she may not be able to resume nursing her child. Having made the recommendation, then, the state may be obligated to provide adequate health education, sterile equipment, clean water, and nutritional formula to prevent unnecessary harm to the children.

Most developing countries lack the resources to ensure safe bottle-feeding for a significant part of their population. Therefore, the policy may have a discriminatory impact. For example, women with sufficient means may be able to safely bottle-feed, but the children of poorer women may become ill, malnourished, or die. The state bears a heavy burden to ensure that children thrive and mature.

A selective policy of recommending bottle-feeding only for known HIV-positive women may reduce the risks of vertical transmission of HIV, but it would expose women to stigma and discrimination. Women who bottle-feed their infants and/or attend special government clinics may be marked as infected with HIV. This distinction may place them and their children at considerable risk of denunciation, particularly in male-dominated societies. In many cultures, the social and economic status of women is closely tied to their male partners and to the woman's fertility. If partners reject women because of their HIV status, or if their ability to bear and raise healthy babies is questioned, they may be shunned by their families and communities or abandoned without a means of support.

Search for a range of less restrictive alternatives

Whenever policies burden human rights, officials have an obligation to search for a range of less restrictive but equally effective alternatives. In this case, a realistic alternative would be to offer or provide women with full information. The Ministry could advise women of the risk of HIV transmission through breast-feeding and offer to test them on a confidential and voluntary basis. Similarly, the Ministry could advise women of the risks of bottle-feeding. Women could then make an informed choice based upon their assessment of the risks, cultural traditions, and available resources.

Additionally, the Ministry could recommend one or more of the following, some of which are mutually exclusive (1) breast-feeding mothers should avoid initial feeding with colostrum because it may increase the risk of HIV transmission; (2) women known to be uninfected should undertake wet nursing; (3) women should wean their infants earlier to curtail breast-feeding; or (4) women should continue to breast-feed to stimulate their infant's production of potentially protective antibodies (Nicoll, 1993).

In the end, the Ministry of Health simply may not possess sufficient scientific data with which to formulate a policy that is most effective and least burdensome on human rights. The scientific community does not yet know the precise level of risk posed by breast-feeding, the factors that may heighten or lower that risk, and the health impact of artificial feeding in different societies (Ziegler, 1993). Some researchers argue that the only way to obtain accurate information for policy formulation is to conduct randomized trials of breast-fed and bottle-fed infants (Centers for Disease Control and Prevention, 1993a). The next part of this case study uses the Human Rights Impact Assessment to examine such a randomized clinical trial.

International Collaborative Research Involving a Randomized Trial of Breast- and Bottle-feeding

A prestigious research institution in a developed country approaches a small developing country to conduct a clinical trial of the relative risks of HIV transmission to breast- and bottle-fed children. Researchers plan to assign known HIV-positive women in the country to either the bottle-feeding or breast-feeding arm of the study. The researchers would follow both groups for two years in an attempt to determine the added risk of vertical transmission of HIV infection through breast-feeding. In the developed country, approximately sixty to seventy percent of mothers bottle-feed their infants. In the developing country, five to ten percent of all mothers currently bottle-feed their infants. The government and researchers in the developing country agree to the collaborative research. An Institutional Review Board in the developed country undertakes a thorough ethical review of the study, but no comparable review occurs in the developing country.

Assessment: analyze the facts

A threshold question is whether a randomized intervention trial could be conducted at all under contemporary international ethical standards. Guideline 11 of the CIOMS (1993) International Ethical Guidelines on Biomedical Research addresses pregnant or nursing women as research subjects. The guidelines do not prohibit research that "carries no more than minimal risk to the fetus or nursing infant" and is "designed to protect or advance the health of pregnant or nursing women or fetuses or nursing infants."

If this trial were conducted in a setting where a substantial proportion of mothers used artificial feeding, it would create significant ethical problems. HIV-positive women who normally would bottle-feed their infants could be randomized to a breast-feeding group, risking the infant's exposure to HIV. Many research ethicists in the international community might view this risk as unacceptable.

If the trial were conducted in a setting where a substantial proportion of mothers breast-fed, significant ethical dilemmas also arise, imposing obligations on the researchers. The initial ethical question is whether it would be culturally feasible to assign mothers in the community to a bottle-feeding group. Would these women accept bottle-feeding and randomization?

The researchers would be obliged to supply health education, sterile equipment, clean water, and other health services to protect the bottle-fed infants from exposure to additional risks of infections, diarrheal disease, or malnutrition. International ethical standards require researchers to minimize all risks to research subjects (CIOMS, 1991, 1993; World Medical Association, 1964).

Although ethically necessary, providing services to mothers and infants to reduce morbidity and mortality from other causes may limit the study's utility. The study should provide useful data on the additional risks of HIV infection from breast-feeding. However, the research cannot answer the more important question of which practice (e.g., breast- or bottle-feeding) produces better overall outcomes for infants and mothers. Therefore, the ethical and human rights implications of undertaking the trial differ from those of a policy that discourages some mothers from breast-feeding (see above, A Policy of Artificial Feeding for an Entire or Select Population; Centers for Disease Control and Prevention, 1993a).

If the study were conducted, how might it be ethically designed and conducted? CIOMS (1993) asks whether international collaborative research addresses a pressing health problem in the host country. Developing countries with high prevalence of HIV and high rates of breast-feeding clearly have a strong interest in understanding the attributable risk of breast-feeding. However, the issue is far more complex. If the study reveals a significantly elevated risk from breast-feeding, it still may not alter public health advice, practices, or traditions in the country. If a mother in the poorest community relies on the study's new data, does she have a viable alternative to breast-feeding? If women lack the resources to be tested for HIV and to be educated in the safe use of formula-feeding, then the study has not benefitted them or their community. For such a study to take place, therefore, a plan should be devised to help the community gain the benefits of the research. If this cannot be accomplished, the study might be more appropriately conducted in a country that could support formula-feeding for a significant part of its infected population.

Examine the public health interest

As discussed above, the public health interest of the research is valid and important in communities where mothers breast-feed their infants. Discovering the attributable risk from breast-feeding may be seen as the first in a series of research steps that lead to lowering infant mortality.

Examine the overall effectiveness of the research

A randomized intervention trial is one of the most effective research methods for understanding public health problems. Despite the ethical problems, a well-designed study would likely answer significant public health questions about vertical transmission of HIV.

Examine the issue of consent

Special efforts to obtain informed consent are necessary in research-naive communities with low educational levels, high illiteracy rates, and cultural and language differences. Adequate and culturally relevant educational efforts are important to inform the research subjects and to orient the community at-large. Research must explain the nature and purpose of the study to subjects in comprehensible language. Possible risks to the mother (e.g., breaches of privacy, discrimination, inability to change to breast-feeding after initial bottle-feeding, increased fertility in non–breast-feeding participants) and to the infant (e.g., malnutrition and disease) must be discussed in the local language using concepts relevant to the social setting.

To assure that research participants are adequately "compensated" without being coerced, incentives for participation, recruitment, and retention will require sensitivity to the specific economic and social norms in the community. For example, in some communities in sub-Saharan Africa, accepting a gift of money may be culturally inappropriate. Instead, researchers might consider granting a small loan to help a subject set up a business, or giving a gift of health care or food.

Determine the impact on human rights

Participation in intervention research of this kind can burden human rights. These risks must be understood and ameliorated. Researchers have a duty to protect the health and life of research subjects. Accordingly, they must consider providing routine health care. For subjects who become infected with HIV during the course of the study, specialized care should be available. International ethical guidelines require instituting an appropriate research safety and monitoring board. Ethical issues include prior scientific review of the protocol and early stopping rules.

Confidentiality and Privacy. Research subjects are concerned with maintaining privacy. Safeguards need to be established to protect the confidentiality of information obtained in the course of the research. Some states may have legal requirements to report HIV-infected individuals to the public health department. Such reporting may conflict with patient confidentiality and may serve as a disincentive to participation in breast-feeding trials. Also, simple participation in the research itself sometimes affects personal privacy. Persons who appear at research clinics, receive home visits from investigators, or bottle-feed their infants may be identified as having HIV disease.

Discrimination. Being publicly identified as a person who is living with HIV or AIDS may result in discrimination by employers, landlords, family, and friends. As discussed previously, discrimination against women in male-dominated societies can fundamentally threaten their social, economic, and familial positions.

Principle of Distributive Justice. Collaborating research partners can minimize human rights burdens by thinking through distributive justice principles, the role of ethical review committees, and the development of research and health care infrastructures. Distributive justice in research requires an equitable sharing of benefits and burdens. Host communities bear the burdens of research and deserve a fair share in its gains. Partners in international collaborative research need to arrive at a mutual understanding on this matter. They need to discuss the availability of infant formulas, supplemental feeding services, and health education to individual participants and/or community members after the research is completed. For example, will HIV-infected women who participate in the trial be supported by supplemental feeding services during subsequent pregnancies?

Ethical Review Committees. CIOMS (1991, 1993) recommends that both the sponsoring and the host country perform a full ethical and scientific review of the research. Ethical review in a sponsoring country alone is not likely to consider all the culturally specific harms that may arise. Attention must be given to the risks of breaches of confidentiality, to the potential for discrimination, to cultural norms regarding subject consent, and to permission of elders or community consensus. Consideration should also be given to local and national ethical norms regarding research on women, infants, adolescents, military populations, institutionalized persons, or public welfare recipients.

Development of Research and Health Care Infrastructure. Special incentives may be needed in international collaborative research to compensate local, institutional, and national government participation. Helping to develop infrastructures in host countries can be an effective way to provide incentives and benefits. Host countries can richly contribute both to local public health needs and to research objectives if their scientists and health care professionals obtain the resources, training, and capacity to function as equal partners. Sponsoring countries can contribute through providing high-quality training and education, laboratory and other vital equipment, and prevention and health care services.

Developing strong infrastructures provides support and stability as host countries work to meet ongoing public health and scientific needs. Collaborative research promotes ongoing relationships. A sound infrastructure that endures through lengthy studies and facilitates future research is an important component of international public health planning and research.

Search for a range of less restrictive alternatives

Researchers could explore the possibility of performing studies where a substantial proportion of mothers already use artificial-feeding. Studies could investigate the relationship between artificial-feeding and infant mortality using cohort or case-control approaches. Observational studies will become much more effective as technology improves to allow early, reliable, and cost-effective detection of HIV infection in infants.

CASE STUDY 3: THE POWER OR DUTY TO INFORM SEXUAL OR NEEDLE-SHARING PARTNERS OF THE RISK OF TRANSMISSION[3]

A Hospital Policy Recommending Disclosure to Partners

A twenty-three-year-old married woman, who has a four-year-old daughter, visits a local city hospital for a routine gynecological consultation. During a careful clinical examination, the doctor notes signs of an opportunistic infection that may be associated with HIV infection. The patient consents to a test for HIV, which is performed.

When the patient returns to the doctor's office to obtain the results, the doctor notes that the patient's arms are bruised and that her jaw is slightly swollen. The doctor in-

3. Professor Karen Rothenberg developed the ideas for this case study for a conference on tuberculosis organized by the U.S. Agency for Health Care Policy and Research in Miami, 1993.

forms the patient that the HIV test was positive and suggests that the patient tell her husband. The woman resists. The doctor explains that the husband is at a significant risk of HIV infection through sexual intercourse and that testing him could have clinical benefits and could lead to safer behaviors. The patient is adamant; she does not want to tell him. She confides that her husband physically abuses her and that she fears that discussing the test results with him will escalate the violence. In addition, she states that she dreads that her husband may divorce her, because he wants a wife who will bear and raise a healthy son. Furthermore, she believes that her husband might seek custody of their daughter, and that her larger family and community will reject her. The doctor sympathizes, but nonetheless urges the woman to reconsider, given the high risk of HIV transmission and the magnitude of the likely harm.

The doctor waits several months, but when she does not hear from the husband, she concludes that her patient has not informed him of the test results. The doctor contacts an elder member of the patient's family to discuss the dilemma: Should she tell the husband that he is at high risk of HIV infection, although she knows that the patient opposes this and faces potential physical and other dangers? Soon thereafter, the husband learns about the test results. As expected, he severely beats his wife, calls her an unfit mother, banishes her from the home, and retains custody of their daughter.

Assessment

The city hospital has no formal policy to direct a health care worker who has knowledge that a patient is infected with HIV. Studies suggest that the low seroprevalence in the heterosexual population is increasing. The hospital is considering whether to introduce a policy that would require doctors to inform the sexual and needle-sharing partners of known HIV-infected patients.

Analyze the facts

Here, the hospital and doctor face an increasingly common dilemma: The doctor possesses knowledge obtained in the course of a confidential relationship with a patient; a patient's apparent sexual partner appears to be at significant risk of exposure to HIV infection; and the patient is at risk of violence from that individual (North, Rothenberg, 1993). To assess this situation, the doctor needs more information about the marital relationship. Is the patient presently engaging in sexual intercourse with her husband or others? Is the husband using a condom and following public health recommendations for safer sex? Is the husband aware that he may have been exposed to HIV, and does he know or have reason to know his serological status? Is he having sex or sharing drug injection equipment outside the marriage, potentially exposing others to HIV?

By disclosing the information to the husband, the doctor might avert a significant and preventable risk to him. Even if the spouse were already infected with HIV, he could seek treatment and counseling to avoid high-risk behaviors. If he were not infected, he could use safer sex techniques with his wife to avoid contracting the infection. On the other hand, disclosure may place the patient at significant risk of ostracism, discrimination, and physical harm.

Examine the public health interest

The hospital should clearly and narrowly define the policy's public health objective to protect against biases in policymaking and to guide health care workers in their practices. Informing a sexual or needle-sharing partner of the risk of HIV infection encompasses several valid objectives. Individuals who are unaware of the risk of infection can seek testing and counseling; discussions with professional counselors can facilitate treatment and support. The person can also use this information to modify behaviors that pose a risk of transmitting the virus.

Examine the overall effectiveness of the policy

This step requires one to assess whether informing sexual or needle-sharing partners is an effective and appropriate means of achieving the stated objectives. The policy's primary goal is to prevent HIV transmission among sexual and needle-sharing partners.

The following scenario presents the most compelling case for informing the husband: He is unaware of his serological status and engages in ongoing sexual relationships and/or needle sharing within or outside the marriage. The knowledge that he may have been exposed to HIV, together with professional counseling, could promote behavioral changes necessary to prevent further transmission of HIV infection.

Despite the policy's potential effectiveness, health care workers must recognize the possible unintended public health effects. Divulging a patient's HIV status to a sexual partner can result in significant harms. This case illustrates the most blatant harm—physical abuse by one's spouse. Moreover, the disclosure here disrupted a parent–child relationship, separating a mother from her preschool-aged daughter. Less obvious harms may be just as devastating. For instance, the wife may be ejected from the household, and possibly left homeless and without financial support. Her family and community may ostracize, shame, and discriminate against her. Health care workers must carefully weigh these tangible harms.

The policy may actually undermine the objective of preventing HIV transmission in the community. If persons at risk for HIV are aware of the policy and feel that their confidences may be betrayed, they may be reluctant to visit the hospital or clinic and may decline testing or withhold important information from health care workers and counselors.

Examine the issue of consent

The policy is being implemented without the patient's consent. In this case, the patient not only refuses to grant consent to disclose the information but has powerful reasons for doing so. She is competent to assess the benefits and risks of disclosure, and chooses to maintain the confidentiality of this information. The hospital would need to show a significant risk of substantial harm to others before overriding the informed decision of a competent adult.

Evaluate whether the policy is well-targeted

Initially, the hospital policy appears well targeted because only those persons at significant risk of exposure will be informed. Yet, the hospital could further narrow the focus by allowing the patient a clear opportunity to disclose the information herself, by requiring an ongoing sexual relationship to prevent *prospective* harms, and by assessing whether the sexual partner has reason to believe that he may have been exposed to HIV (For policy alternatives that might protect the patient's confidentiality and warn the partner of possible sexual exposure, see below, Search for a Range of Less Restrictive Alternatives).

Determine the impact on human rights

This step requires inquiry into the nature, invasiveness, scope, and duration of human rights violations. The hospital policy substantially burdens the right to privacy. To disclose a patient's HIV status, even if only to partners, divulges information about health as well as intimate personal conduct. This information may, for example, reveal a person's infidelity or injecting drug use, matters that may destroy a relationship. Furthermore, the partner has no formal duty to maintain confidentiality, and may disclose the intimate information to others in the family, village, or community.

In this case, the doctor first disclosed the information to an elder family member. While possibly consistent with local traditions and norms, this nonetheless constitutes a breach of trust. The information then found its way to the patient's partner, who severely battered her.

Unwarranted breaches of confidentiality may deeply burden a patient's right to free association by interfering with complex personal relationships. The policy may even threaten family unity, as in this case; members may reject a person who has HIV infection at the time when she most needs support. A spouse may retaliate by removing the children from the home, depriving them of a parent's care, rejecting the woman, and/or refusing to provide her with financial support. Such interferences may have lifelong consequences for persons living with HIV infection and may undermine the person's rights to family, health, and, perhaps, life itself.

Persons with HIV infection also risk discrimination in the workplace, health care settings, and the wider community. In cultures where women's social and economic status depend upon their marital and maternal status, women may be at particular risk of discrimination.

Search for a range of less restrictive alternatives

Considering less restrictive alternatives may help to resolve each side's compelling legal and ethical claims. One alternative is to empower vulnerable populations, such as abused women, so that they may better protect themselves physically, socially, and economically; such programs could mitigate the consequences of disclosing HIV information to their partners. For example, the government might modify its divorce and custody laws to protect HIV-infected women from becoming abandoned, impoverished, or deprived of their children. Social programs and legal reform are constructive long-term steps to reduce the social impact of HIV. Such action, however, still might not sufficiently protect an individual from harm.

A better option might be to adopt partner notification programs modeled on those traditionally used in the field of public health for sexually transmitted infections (STIs). Here, the public health department, not the health care worker, has the duty to inform sexual partners. Partner notification programs traditionally protect human rights while safeguarding the public health: The person with the STI is not coerced into releasing partners' names; he or she must give informed consent for disclosure; and the partner is not given the name of the person who may have exposed them to the infection. Moreover, public health officials have discretion regarding whether to inform the partner. This enables the official to examine each individual case with flexibility and to determine whether the harm to the person with the STI outweighs the benefit of disclosure. A real threat of violence might caution against wielding the power to warn persons at significant risk.

Determine whether the policy meets the significant risk standard

If the administrator concludes that imposing a duty to warn is the least restrictive and most effective approach, he or she should undertake an individualized determination of whether a person with HIV infection poses a significant risk to others. The policy should also undergo a careful evaluation of its potential harms. The latter step might have prevented the doctor from disclosing her patient's HIV status to a family elder; the doctor had observed evidence of physical abuse and knew that her patient had not consented to notifying the husband. Here, the following factors might outweigh the spouse's right to know: the lack of effective biomedical interventions, the likelihood of violence against the patient, disruption of the family, social stigmatization, and other unintended consequences. If the significant risk standard is met, a health care worker should try to obtain the patient's consent by listening to her concerns and discussing the issues with sensitivity.

A Law Granting a Broad Range of Individuals a "Right to Know" if They May Have Been Exposed to HIV

The press reports this story, depicting the husband as the victim of a sexually promiscuous wife. The lawmaking body decides to hold hearings on whether to enact a broad "right to know" statute that would require persons exposed to HIV to be informed. The right would apply to persons who may have been exposed to HIV through spitting, biting, physical assault, sexual intercourse, needle sharing, caring for a person with HIV infection, or handling the body of a deceased AIDS patient. Public health authorities would notify these persons (e.g., sexual or needle-sharing partners; health care, emergency, and mortuary workers; assault victims; school officials; and others with whom the person might have come in contact) of their potential exposure, and would identify the person with HIV. Should the legislature enact such a statute?

Assessment: analyze the facts

To analyze the proposed policy from both a public health and human rights perspective, the legislature must objectively examine the facts. Policymakers should collect information from a variety of credible sources and rely only on scientifically sound data. Consulting multiple sources and maintaining high scientific standards help to protect against biases or acquiescence to popular fears.

Medical and scientific data do not support the need for such a broad statute. Current scientific information limits the recognized modes of HIV transmission to sexual intercourse, the use of contaminated injection equipment, exposure to infected blood products, and vertical transmission from mother to child during pregnancy, birth, and lactation. These modes constitute the only scientifically defensible basis for broad-reaching public health policies to prevent HIV infections. No evidence exists that HIV can be transmitted through routine contact between a person with HIV infection and health care or emergency workers, school personnel, or most others contemplated by the statute. Even where exposure is possible, such as during some health care procedures, no data indicate that knowing the HIV status of the patient will protect the worker (see Chapter 4: The Health Care System). Enacting a policy that grants such a vast array of persons a right to know could perpetuate and reinforce the unfounded fear that HIV can be spread through casual contact.

The proposed policy also reflects the misguided belief that persons with HIV infection are likely to expose others intentionally to the virus. No evidence suggests that this is a common phenomenon. The majority of persons with HIV act responsibly. In fact, persons with HIV/AIDS have designed and implemented some of the most effective prevention and education programs (United Nations, 1991).

Examine the public health interest

When lawmakers react to a publicized individual case, they must clearly and carefully define their public health objectives. This helps to ensure that policies are based on a compelling public health interest rather than prejudices, stereotypes, or irrational fears.

In this case, if the purpose of the statute is to prevent HIV transmission, it is vague and overbroad. Although most HIV policies ultimately seek this as their purpose, a more narrowly described objective is needed to evaluate the policy's effectiveness and impact. Policymakers could claim that the objective is to inform people who "might be" or have been exposed to HIV infection. But this interest, as defined by the statute, does not appear to be compelling. The proposed law includes some "exposures" (e.g., spitting, biting, and physical assault) that pose only the most remote risk of transmission. Similarly, persons to be informed include those whose risk of exposure is minimal (e.g., health care workers and school personnel). Preventing remote risks to persons unlikely to be exposed is not a compelling interest. The policy may also conflict with the locality or country's priorities, since it could consume considerable resources while failing to address more prevalent modes of transmission.

A second objective—warning those who have been intentionally exposed—is not compelling either, because no evidence suggests that intentional exposure is a common or likely mode of transmission. Absent such evidence, most jurisdictions could not consider this objective as a priority.

The policy's goal is most compelling if it aims to inform people who currently are at a real or substantial risk of HIV infection but are otherwise unlikely to know that they may have been exposed. As written, the proposed statute is much broader than this relatively narrow description (see below, Evaluate Whether the Policy Is Well-Targeted; Search for a Range of Less Restrictive Alternatives).

Examine the overall effectiveness of the policy

Even a compelling objective does not necessarily justify a "right to know" law. The legislature should evaluate whether the policy is an appropriate intervention to achieve the objectives and whether it is reasonably likely to be effective.

Here, disclosing the identity of HIV-infected individuals to this range of people must further the stated goal. In some cases, knowing that a sexual or needle-sharing partner has HIV infection could lead a person to alter behavior to prevent infection. However, experience in the area of HIV prevention and education programs indicates that knowledge of HIV status alone does not bring about lasting behavioral changes necessary to prevent transmission. Counseling, education, and accessible means of protection are necessary to effect such changes. The policy does not, on its face, provide these critical elements. In low-risk settings, such as hospitals, knowledge of patients' HIV status has not prevented accidental exposure of health care workers to HIV by contaminated needles or sharp instruments.

This policy will not achieve its objective by warning everyone who might come into contact with persons with HIV infection. Many people will remain undiagnosed. Individuals who fear that their HIV status will be disclosed might not seek testing. Thus, the proportion of undiagnosed cases could increase. A "right to know" policy could also have the unintended effect of increasing exposures if it leads to a false sense of security and people stopped practicing safer sex or other protective measures.

Examine the issue of consent

Legal and ethical standards strongly suggest that public health programs incorporate the principle of informed consent. The policy at issue does not require authorities to obtain the consent of the person with HIV infection before disclosing his or her identity to a potentially large number of people. Earlier in this chapter, as A Hospital Policy Recommending Disclosures to Partners demonstrates, an individual may have well-founded reasons to refuse disclosure, and disclosure without her consent may lead to serious harm. The proposed law has no provision for authorities to seek consent or to evaluate the reasons for refusal. This omission indicates a lack of respect for the individual's capacity to weigh the risks and benefits and to make a responsible decision. Authorities should view the process of informed consent as a dialogue in which both the patient and the provider exchange relevant information. Together, they then could determine whether disclosure is warranted as either necessary or beneficial in the particular situation.

Weigh the opportunity costs

By implementing a right-to-know policy, lawmakers may forgo other more cost-effective programs. The resources required to implement and enforce this policy could restrict or eliminate prevention and education programs, voluntary and confidential partner notification programs, and perhaps even programs to help battered women. Adoption of this policy might also reduce public pressure on lawmakers to establish more effective programs, because people might believe that they are somehow protected by the right to know.

Evaluate whether the policy is well-targeted

The proposed legislation is overinclusive. It grants a broad right to know to persons who come in casual contact with individuals who have HIV. Since casual contact poses no risk of transmission, and spitting, biting, and physical assault pose very little risk, the policy would unduly disclose sensitive information to more people than it would actually benefit. Since the policy does not limit disclosure to current or prospective exposures, it could apply to persons who long ago had a relationship or even minor contact with the HIV-infected person. Moreover, the policy would disclose the identity of the person with HIV infection to others even if these persons knew they had been exposed to HIV from another source. Furthermore, the policy seems to assume that persons with HIV infection will not voluntarily inform others who may be at risk, and that they will not modify their own behavior to protect others.

In addition to being overinclusive, this policy also may be underinclusive. It will not reach individuals who avoid HIV testing out of fear of disclosure or those who may expose others because they lack the education and counseling that a voluntary system can provide. Authorities may target certain populations assumed to engage in "risky behaviors" or to have a higher risk of HIV infection. Singling out individuals or groups in this context unjustifiably discriminates against them, exposes them to stigmatization, and reinforces stereotypes about the epidemic.

Determine the impact on human rights

Even a narrowly tailored policy to achieve a compelling public health purpose should be weighed against its potential human rights burdens. Sometimes, substantial public health benefits will justify infringements on human rights. Where the public health objective is less than compelling, however, or poorly targeted, human rights burdens may tip the balance against implementation. In assessing infringements on human rights, policymakers should consider their nature, invasiveness, scope, and duration.

The first part of this case illustrated how a policy authorizing disclosure without an individual's consent substantially infringes on privacy and the related principles of confidentiality and informed consent. Disclosure of an individual's HIV status without her consent is extremely intrusive; it reveals highly personal information and can lead to destructive inferences and actions by others. Involuntary disclosure is warranted only to protect others from imminent and probable harm. As case study 1 demonstrated, revealing HIV status to persons who face a theoretical or remote risk of infection is not justified.

The number of persons affected by this policy and the frequency of human rights violations would be considerable. On its face, the policy applies to all persons with HIV infection, regardless of whether they themselves agree to notify their partners. The policy also authorizes disclosure to many people who interact with each infected person. Since no confidentiality obligation binds persons who are informed as part of this policy, they may further disclose the sensitive information to the infected person's family, friends, employers, and insurers. As a result, the person with HIV infection could lose her housing, employment, insurance, children, and her family's emotional and financial support. She may be discriminated against, stigmatized, or ostracized by individuals and the community.

In addition to the rights of privacy and equal treatment, such broad-based disclosure could unjustifiably burden the right to health by denying persons with HIV infection medical insurance or prompting health care workers to refuse treatment. It could also infringe on the right to family unity by denying persons with HIV infection equal rights to custody of their children or by establishing a basis for unfavorable divorce terms. This policy could inflict life-long pain, suffering, and deprivation on HIV-infected individuals.

Search for a range of less restrictive alternatives

A critical step in evaluating a policy that infringes on human rights is to determine whether other policies might achieve the public health objective as effectively while imposing fewer human rights burdens. The principle of the least restrictive alternative recommends adoption of the least intrusive, equally effective alternative.

The legislature should first consider voluntary approaches. A prevention and education program that encourages persons at risk of infection to seek counseling and testing and provides access to harm reduction strategies (such as condoms and clean needles) respects human rights and could lead to lasting behavior changes. Confidential notification through the health department with the consent of HIV-infected persons would enable authorities to warn most of the individuals at significant risk of infection, would preserve the trust between health care providers and patients, and would not burden human rights. If policymakers remain concerned about warning those who do not know that they are at risk, they might, as another alternative, grant public health authorities the power, but not the duty, to warn an unsuspecting partner when all other measures have failed.

To ensure use of the least restrictive alternative in each case, lawmakers could adopt a policy with a series of steps for warning persons at substantial risk of infection. The policy could require medical and public health officials to begin with entirely voluntary measures. Only if these measures were unsuccessful would the policy authorize the use of coercion or the disclosure of information without a patient's consent. Additionally, authorities should rigorously evaluate all the risks and benefits of disclosure and attempt to mitigate any harms that result from these judgments.

Determine whether the policy meets the significant risk standard and provides fair procedures

This step requires a case-by-case determination of the risks actually posed by a particular individual. Granting broad classes of persons the right to know, without reference to individual situations, is troubling.

Although HIV is incurable, the severity of harm alone does not prove that a significant risk exists. To establish a significant risk, lawmakers should demonstrate not only grave harm but also the real possibility and probability of transmission, and the continuity of risk.

As we saw above, many of the modes of transmission recognized in the statute (such as spitting, biting, and physical assault) pose little or no risk of infection. Similarly, the probability of transmission to certain persons (such as health care providers, emergency workers, and school personnel) is remote. The significance of the risk depends upon the facts of each case. Given the objective scientific data about transmission, policymakers would likely fail to show that routine contact poses a significant risk of infection.

The significant risk test may be satisfied in situations involving sexual or needle-sharing partners: The harm is serious, the modes of transmission are well established, and the duration of the risk is life-long. Furthermore, the probability of harm may be substantial if sexual intercourse or needle sharing is ongoing, if the other partner is not yet infected, or if neither partner uses safety precautions. To establish that a person with HIV infection poses a significant risk to her sexual or needle-sharing partners, authorities must know more about the relationship than the HIV status of one partner.

Consequently, fair procedures would include requiring public health authorities to evaluate all the risks and benefits of disclosure and allowing them to withhold confidential information when the harms outweigh the potential benefits.

Afterword

The discovery of connections between human rights and HIV/AIDS was very intense, emotional, and personal. At the World Health Organization, starting in 1986, reports were received that HIV-infected people and people with AIDS were suffering specific forms of discrimination: in the workplace, in schools, in travel, and in health care. These discriminatory actions were not occurring in any single country, or social setting, or culture or religion: tragic human stories of rejection, denial, and even violence were brought to our attention by colleagues from around the world. And, most poignantly, in the words of many people with AIDS, that stigmatization and abandonment by others was felt as even more cruel than the fact of disease, or impending death itself.

Therefore, at WHO, we started a process of refusal of discrimination directed towards HIV-infected people and people with AIDS (well described in this book) which has led, ultimately, to major changes in how public health defines itself and to a new movement which links health and human rights inextricably together.

This process, representing a profound professional evolution, can be roughly divided into three stages. The first stage focused on recognizing and responding to discrimination directed against already HIV-infected people. The need to prevent such discrimination resulted both from its evident unfairness and cruelty, as well as from an analysis of its public health consequences. For we discovered that when people became afraid to discover if they were HIV-infected, due to justified fear of severe personal and social consequences (loss of job, expulsion from school, prohibition of marriage), people no longer sought to learn their HIV infection status. The resulting decline in HIV testing thereby undermined public health efforts to help prevent the spread of HIV. Thus, a public health rationale for preventing discrimination towards HIV-infected people and people with AIDS was developed, and it became an integral part of the Global AIDS Strategy. For the first time in history, preventing discrimination towards infected people was part of a strategy to control an epidemic disease.

The first phase therefore considered discrimination as a tragic and counter-productive "effect" of the HIV/AIDS pandemic. In the second phase, it became apparent that the lack of respect for human rights and dignity was also a profoundly important "root cause" of vulnerability to the pandemic.

This second phase of discovery arose as we realized that the HIV/AIDS pandemic was evolving in a particular direction in each society. That is, it became clear that those populations who, before AIDS arrived, were already societally marginalized or stigmatized, became at greatest risk of HIV infection. Thus, in every society, while the early history of the epidemic may have been very different (initially involving, for example, injection drug users, or people with hemophilia, or women sex workers or gay men), with time, those already discriminated against within the society gradually came to bear the brunt of the epidemic. This helped to understand why, for example, married and monogamous women in various societies were becoming HIV-infected; they could not refuse unwanted or unprotected sexual intercourse with their husbands, even if they knew he was HIV-infected, because they lacked the social status and rights which could protect them. Very concretely, refusal of sexual intercourse could result in being beaten, with no civil recourse, or to being divorced (unilaterally decided by the man), which, because the woman would have no rights to property, would lead to a condition equivalent to civil and economic death for the woman. Thus, through these analyses in various countries and settings, it became evident that the status of respect for human rights and dignity defined the level of societal vulnerability to HIV/AIDS. This insight was articulated at WHO in the late 1980s and was developed further by the Global AIDS Policy Coalition (an independent, multidisciplinary AIDS advocacy group created in 1991) in its book, "AIDS in the World" (1992).

Thus, the second phase in this discovery process identified vulnerability to HIV as resulting from a lack of respect for, or realization of human rights and dignity. In turn this led to a series of efforts to improve the ability of AIDS workers to identify and respond to the human rights implications of their work, and to understand why and how improving the status of human rights was essential for progress against the HIV pandemic. An example of this work, referred to extensively in this book, was the manual entitled "AIDS, Health and Human Rights," produced by the International Federation of Red Cross and Red Crescent Societies and the François-Xavier Bagnoud Center for Health and Human Rights at Harvard.

It has been very exciting to see that the new UNAIDS program has adopted this perspective—explicitly linking promotion of human rights with prevention of HIV infection—in its philosophy and work plans.

On the personal level, after resigning as director of the Global Program on AIDS at WHO in 1990, the opportunity arose, in the context of moving to an academic institution, to broaden lessons from AIDS to health more generally. Rather than seeing HIV/ AIDS as an exception, we examined other health issues—from heart disease, to maternal mortality, to injuries and domestic violence—and realized that the same basic principle seemed to apply. Namely, that the vulnerability of people to these health problems seemed integrally connected to the status of realization of their human rights. The history of women's health was particularly relevant, for earlier work had demonstrated clearly how women's reproductive health was intricately linked with the level of respect for women's reproductive rights. Indeed, the World Bank, not generally considered a human rights advocate, identified (in the World Development Report—1993) increased realization of women's rights to education as one of the most powerful interventions to improve health in the developing world!

We developed these insights, born from earlier work in women's health and from experience in the human rights dimensions of HIV/AIDS, and proposed a three-part provisional framework for thinking more broadly about the relationship between health and human rights.

First, public health policies or programs may burden or even violate human rights; in response, we developed a method (also described in this book) to negotiate an optimal balance between achieving public health goals and respecting human rights norms.

Second, all human rights violations have impacts on health, particularly when the WHO definition of health as "physical, mental and social well-being" is applied. In response, we began to identify and map out how violations of a wide range of civil and political, as well as economic and social rights lead to adverse health effects.

Third, we articulated the concept that promoting and protecting health is inextricably linked with promoting and protecting health. We have stated that modern human rights provides a better framework for analyzing and responding to the societal dimensions of health than any framework or method inherited from the biomedical or public health tradition. Thus, we have called upon health professionals and human rights advocates to work together to identify how and where the lack of respect for human rights leads to preventable illnesses, disabilities, and premature death. We have identified human rights as the best description available of the societal conditions in which people can achieve the optimal state of health; from this point forward, the goals of public health cannot be separated from the goal of improving realization of human rights and respect for human dignity around the world.

In 1993, the François-Xavier Bagnoud Center for Health and Human Rights, the first academic center to focus exclusively on the connection between health and human rights, was created at Harvard. Since that time, two International Conferences on Health and Human Rights have been held, a new journal ("Health and Human Rights") serves as a forum for discussion of health and human rights issues, and an increasing number of educational courses at schools of public health around the world have been launched. A global movement linking health and human rights, and revitalizing the field of public health as well as challenging the traditional practices of human rights, is now well underway.

Gostin and Lazzarini have performed a very useful service to us all, bringing together information about health and human rights in the context of HIV/AIDS. This description of the expanding field of health and human rights is most welcome, for it has been through the experience of HIV/AIDS that we have come to recognize how human rights, more than medical care or any other factor, affects our health; that human rights and dignity determine to a large extent, who shall live and who shall die, when, and of what. Now we are learning how to act on this vital insight, which opens a new era in the history of health and society.

Jonathan M. Mann, M.D., M.P.H.
François-Xavier Bagnoud Professor
of Health and Human Rights, Harvard School of Public Health

Bibliography

HUMAN RIGHTS DOCUMENTS

International

Alston P. (1993) *Human Rights in 1993: How Far Has the United Nations Come and Where Should It Go From Here?* Paper presented at the International Conference on Human Rights, Vienna, 14–25 June 1993.

American Association for the Advancement of Science. (1993) *Socio-Economic Indicators and Human Rights*. Background paper presented to the seminar on appropriate indicators to measure achievements in the progressive realization of economic, social and cultural rights, Geneva, 25–29 January 1993. HR/GENEVA/1993/SEM/BP.1.

Committee for Development Planning. (1993) *A Note on Indicators of Economic and Social Rights*. Background paper presented to the seminar on appropriate indicators to measure achievements in the progressive realization of economic, social and cultural rights, Geneva, 25–29 January 1993. HR/GENEVA/1993/SEM/BP.9.

Council of International Organizations of Medical Sciences (CIOMS). (1991) *International Guidelines for Ethical Review of Epidemiological Studies*. CIOMS, Geneva.

Council of International Organizations of Medical Sciences (CIOMS). (1993) *International Ethical Guidelines for Biomedical Research Involving Human Subjects*. CIOMS, Geneva.

International Health Regulations. (1985) International health regulation (1969). *Weekly Epidemiological Record* 60:311, October 4, 1985.

International Slavery Convention. (1926)

Nuremberg Code. (1947) Printed in *Trials of War Criminals Before the Nuremberg Military Tribunals Under Control Council Law No. 10* 2:181–182, Washington, DC: U.S. Government Printing Office, 1949.

Principles of Medical Ethics. (1982) Resolution adopted by the United Nations General Assembly, 9 March 1983. A/RES/37/194.

Proclamation of Teheran. (1968)

Siracusa Principles. (1984) U.N. Document No. E/CN.4/1984/4.

United Nations. (1959) *Declaration of the Rights of the Child*. U.N. Document No. A/4354/1959.

United Nations. (1984) *The United Nations and Human Rights*. U.N. Sales No. E.84.I.6, New York.

United Nations. (1986) *The Right to Development*. U.N. Document No. A/41/1986/53.

United Nations. (1990) *Freedom of the Individual Under Law: A Study on the Individual's Duties to the Community and the Limitations on Human Rights and Freedoms Under Art. 29 of the Universal Declaration of Human Rights, by Erica-Irene A. Daes, Special Rapporteur*. The Commission on Human Rights, Subcommission on Prevention of Discrimination and Protection of Minorities. U.N. Sales No. E.89.XIV.5, New York.

United Nations. (1990b) *The Rights of Indigenous Peoples.* Centre for Human Rights. United Nations, Geneva.

United Nations. (1991a) *The Protection of Persons with Mental Illness and the Improvement of Mental Health Care.* Resolution No. 46/119, adopted by the General Assembly, 17 December 1991.

United Nations. (1991b) *The Realization of the Right to Development: Global Consultation on the Right to Development as a Human Right.* United Nations, New York.

United Nations. (1992a) *Report on the Sale of Children, by Vitil Muntarbhorn, Special Rapporteur.* The Commission on Human Rights. U.N. Doc. No. E/CN.4/1992/55 and Add.1.

United Nations. (1993a) The Right to Health: Conceptualizing a Minimum Core Content. Working paper presented by Audrey R. Chapman, Director Science and Human Rights Programme, American Association for the Advancement of Science, to the Committee on Economic, Social and Cultural Rights—Implementation of the International Covenant on Economic, Social and Cultural Rights, Geneva, 22 November–10 December 1993. E/C.12/1993/WP.24.

United Nations. (1993b) Implementation of the International Covenant on Economic, Social, and Cultural Rights. Working paper presented by Virginia A. Leary, to the Committee on Economic, Social and Cultural Rights—Implementation of the International Covenant on Economic, Social and Cultural Rights, Geneva, 22 November–10 December 1993. E/C.12/1993/WP.27.

Vienna Declaration and Programme of Action. (1993) Declaration from the United Nations, World Conference on Human Rights. Vienna, 14–25 June 1993. A/CONF.157/23, 12 July 1993.

World Health Organization. (1946) Constitution of the World Health Organization, signed on 22 July 1946 by representatives of the 61 member states. *Official Record of the World Health Organization,* 2, 100.

World Health Organization. (1978) Declaration of Alma Ata. Adopted at the International Conference on Primary Health Care.

World Health Organization. (1982) Council for International Organizations of Medical Sciences. *Proposed International Guidelines for Biomedical Research Involving Human Subjects.* Geneva.

World Health Organization. (1993c) *Human Rights in Relation to Women's Health: The Promotion and Protection of Women's Health through International Human Rights Law.* Prepared by Cook RJ. Geneva, WHO/DGH/93.1.

World Health Organization. (1993d) *Indicators to Measure the Realization of the Right to Health.* Background paper presented to the seminar on appropriate indicators to measure achievements in the progressive realization of economic, social and cultural rights, Geneva, 25–29 January 1993. HR/GENEVA/1993/SEM/BP.19.

World Medical Association. (1964) Declaration of Helsinki: Recommendations Guiding Medical Doctors in Biomedical Research Involving Human Subjects, adopted by the 18th World Medical Assembly, Helsinki, Finland, 1964, revised by the 29th WHA, Tokyo, Japan, 1975, the 35th WHA in Venice, Italy, 1983, and the 41st World Medical Assembly, Hong Kong, September, 1989. Reprinted in Medical Ethics Declarations. *World Medical Journal* 31:4, 1984.

Regional

A. v. United Kingdom (1980) application no. 6840/74. Report of the European Commission of Human Rights, adopted 16 July.

B. v. United Kingdom (1981) application no. 6870/75. Report of the European Commission of Human Rights, adopted 7 October.

Van der Leer v. The Netherlands (1990) The Times, March 2, 1990. European Court of Human Rights.
Winterwerp v. The Netherlands (1979) 2 E.H.R.R. 387. European Court of Human Rights.
X. v. United Kingdom (1981) 4 E.H.R.R. 188. European Court of Human Rights.

National

Americans with Disabilities Act (1990) United States Public Law 101–336.
Commonwealth v. Leno (1993) 415 Mass. 835.
Indian Council of Medical Research. (1980)*Policy Statement on Ethical Considerations Involved in Research on Human Beings.* ICMR, New Delhi.
People v. Bordowitz (1991) 588 N.Y.S.2d 507.
Spokane County Health District v. Brockett (1992) 120 Wash.2d 140.
State v. Sorge (1991) 591 A.2d 1382.
Ware v. Valley Stream High School District (1989) 75 N.Y.2d 114, 551 N.Y.S.2d 167.

AIDS-Specific

American Medical Association. (1996) *Counseling and Testing of Women for HIV.* House of Delegates Resolution number 425, adopted June 27, 1996.
Commonwealth Secretariat. (1990) *Ethical and Social Aspects of AIDS in Africa.* Consultants report by Julia Hausermann. August 1990.
Council of Europe. (1987)*Recommendation N. R. (87) 25 of the Committee of Ministers to Member States on a Common European Health Policy to Fight the Acquired Immunodeficiency Syndrome (AIDS).* Council of Europe, 26 November 1987.
Council of Europe. (1988) *Recommendation 1080: on a coordinated European health policy to prevent the spread of AIDS in prisons.* Parliamentary Assembly of the Council of Europe, 30 June 1988.
Council of Europe. (1989a) *Recommendation No. R (89) 14 of the Committee of Ministers to Member States on the ethical issues of HIV infection in the health care and social settings.* 24 October 1989.
Council of Europe. (1989b) *Recommendation 1116 (1989) on AIDS and human rights.* Parliamentary Assembly, 29 September 1989.
Council of Europe. (1990)*Recommendation No.R(90) 3 concerning medical research on human beings.* Adopted by the Committee of Ministers. 6 February 1990. Human Rights Committee. General Comment 9. CCPR/C/21/Rev.1.
Department of Health, Housing and Community Services. (1992) *The Final Report of the Legal Working Party of the Intergovernmental Committee on AIDS.* Australia, November 1992.
European Parliament. (1989) *Resolution on the fight against AIDS,* Strasbourg, 26 May 1989.
Illinois Department of Public Health. (1989) *Data for the First 12 Months of Mandatory Premarital HIV Testing.* Unpublished report of data showing a 22% decline in the number of marriage licenses obtained in the State of Illinois during 1988.
International Consultation on Health Legislation and Ethics. (1988) *Conclusions and Recommendation of the International Consultation on Health Legislation and Ethics in the Field of AIDS and HIV Infection.* Oslo, 26–29 April 1988.
Merson MH. (1992) *HIV/AIDS, Human Rights and the International Response.* Commission on Human Rights, Sub-Commission on Prevention of Discrimination and Protection of Minorities, Geneva, 21 August 1992.

Office of the General Counsel. (1994) Department of Health and Human Services, Letter of 22 November, Re: Needle Exchange Programs.

Paris Declaration on Women, Children and AIDS. (1989) 27–30 November 1989.

Rights and Humanity Declaration. (1992) Rights and Humanity, International Movement for the Promotion and Realization of Human Rights and Responsibilities. *The Rights and Humanity Declaration and Charter on HIV and AIDS*, the Peace Palace, the Hague, May 1991.

United Nations. (1988) *Prevention and Control of Acquired Immunodeficiency Syndrome (AIDS)*. General Assembly Resolution 43115, 27 October 1988.

United Nations. (1989a) *Prevention and Control of Acquired Immunodeficiency Syndrome (AIDS)*. General Assembly Resolution 44/236, 22 December 1989.

United Nations Centre for Human Rights. (1989b) World Health Organization. *International Consultation on AIDS and Human Rights*. Geneva, 26–28 July 1989. U.N. Doc. HR/AIDS/1989/3.

United Nations. (1989c) *Non-discrimination in the field of health*. Resolution 1989/11 of the Commission on Human Rights of 2 March 1989.

United Nations. (1989d) *Discrimination against HIV-infected people or people with AIDS*. Sub-Commission on the prevention of discrimination and protection of minorities. Resolution 1989/18, 31 August 1989.

United Nations. (1989e) *Possible questions for a study on human rights and AIDS*. Concise notes by Mr. Varela Quiros pursuant to Sub-Commission decision 1988/11. U.N. Doc. E/CN.4/Sub.2/ 1989/5.

United Nations. (1989f) *The effects of AIDS on the advancement of women*. Report of the Secretary-General: conclusions and recommendations. U.N. Doc. E/CN.6/1989/6/Add.1.

United Nations. (1990a) *The Social Context of HIV and Its Effect on Families, Women and Children*. Report of an Expert Group Meeting on Women and HIV/AIDS and the Role of National Machinery for the Advancement of Women, held in Vienna, 24–28 September 1990. Prepared by Alberto Palloni and Yean Ju Lee.

United Nations. (1991) *Discrimination against HIV infected people or people with AIDS: Progress Report by Mr. Luis Varela Quiros, Special Rapporteur*. The Commission on Human Rights, Subcommission on Prevention of Discrimination and Protection of Minorities. 24 July 1991. U.N. Doc. E/CN.4/sub.2/1991/10.

United Nations. (1992) *Discrimination against HIV infected people or people with AIDS: Final Report by Mr. Luis Varela Quiros, Special Rapporteur*. The Commission on Human Rights, Subcommission on Prevention of Discrimination and Protection of Minorities. 28 July 1992. U.N. Doc. E/CN.4/Sub.2/1992/10.

United Nations. (1993) *Discrimination against HIV infected people or people with AIDS Conclusions and Recommendations: Final Report by Mr. Luis Varela Quiros, Special Rapporteur*. The Commission on Human Rights, Subcommission on Prevention of Discrimination and Protection of Minorities. 9 August 1993. U.N. Doc. E/CN.4/Sub.2/1993/9.

United Nations. (1994a) *The protection of human rights in the context of human immunodeficiency virus (HIV) and acquired immunodeficiency syndrome (AIDS)*. Resolution, Commission on Human Rights. 1994/49, 4 March 1994.

United Nations. (1994b) *Discrimination in the context of human immunodeficiency virus (HIV) or acquired immunodeficiency syndrome (AIDS)*. Resolution, Sub-Commission on the Prevention of Discrimination and Protection of Minorities. U.N.Doc.E/CN.4/Sub.2/1994/56, 1994/29. 26 August 1994.

United Nations. (1995a) *The protection of human rights in the context of human immunodeficiency virus (HIV) and acquired immunodeficiency syndrome (AIDS)*. Resolution, Commission on Human Rights. U.N. Doc. RES/HS/95/124, 3 March 1995.

United Nations. (1995b) *Discrimination in the context of human immunodeficiency virus (HIV) or acquired immunodeficiency syndrome (AIDS)*. Resolution, Sub-Commission on the Prevention of Discrimination and Protection of Minorities. U.N. Doc. E/CN.4/Sub.2/1995/L.11/Add.5, 24 August 1995.

United Nations. (1995c) *Report of the Secretary-General on international and domestic measures taken to protect human rights and prevent discrimination in the context of HIV/AIDS*. Commission on Human Rights. U.N. Doc. E/CN.4/1995/45, 22 December 1994.

United Nations. (1995d) *Report of the Special Representative of the Secretary-General on Cambodia, Justice Michael Kirby*. U.N.Doc. E/CN.4/1995/87.

United Nations (UNAIDS). (1995e) *Strategic Plan 1996–2000*. UNAIDS/PCB(2)/95.3.

United Nations (UNAIDS). (1996) *Human Rights and HIV/AIDS*. Statement by Peter Piot, Executive Director UNAIDS, to the Commission on Human Rights, Fifty-second session. Geneva, April 1996.

United Nations. (1996a) *Further Promotion and Encouragement of Human Rights and Fundamental Freedoms, Including the Question of the Programme and Methods of Work of the Commission & Alternative Approaches and Ways and Means Within the United Nations System for Improving the Effective Enjoyment of Fundamental Freedoms*. Report of the Secretary-General on Human Rights and HIV/AIDS. Commission on Human Rights. U.N. Doc. E/CN.4/1996/44, 10 January 1996.

United Nations (UNAIDS). (1996b) *Fact Sheet: Joint United Nations Programme on HIV/AIDS*. May 1996.

United Nations (UNAIDS). (1996c) *HIV/AIDS Surveillance Report*. Geneva. June 6, 1996.

United Nations High Commissioner for Refugees (UNHCR). (1988) *UNHCR health policy on AIDS*. 15 February 1988. UNHCR/IOM/21/88 and UNHCR/FOM/20/88.

United States General Accounting Office. (1993) *Needle Exchange Programs: Research Suggests Promise as an AIDS Strategy*. Washington, DC: U.S. General Accounting Office, 1993.

United States National Commission on AIDS. (1991) *Report: America Living With AIDS: Transforming Anger, Fear and Indifference into Action*. Washington, DC: U.S. Government Printing Office.

World Health Assembly, Fortieth. (1987) *Global Strategy for the Prevention and Control of AIDS*. 15 May 1987. Resolution WHA 40.26.

World Health Assembly, Forty-first. (1988) *Avoidance of discrimination in relation to HIV-infected people and people with AIDS*. Resolution WHA 41.24, 13 May 1988.

World Health Assembly, Forty-second. (1989) *Global Strategy for the Prevention and Control of AIDS*. Resolution WHA 42.33, 19 May 1989.

World Health Assembly, Forty-fifth. (1992) *Global Strategy for Prevention and Control of AIDS*. Resolution WHA 45.35, 14 May 1992.

World Health Assembly, Forty-sixth. (1993) *World Health Assembly calls for elimination of harmful practices*. Press release. Geneva, 12 May 1993.

World Health Organization. (1987a) *Social Aspects of AIDS Prevention and Control Programmes*. WHO Special Programme on AIDS, Geneva, 1 December 1987, WHO/SPA/GLO/87.2.

World Health Organization. (1987b) Special Programme on AIDS statement: *Transmission of HIV, Third meeting of WHO collaborating centres on AIDS*, Washington, 6 June 1987, WHO/SPA/RDV/87.1.

World Health Organization. (1987c) *Criteria that must be considered in planning and implementing HIV screening programmes*—Report of the WHO meeting on criteria for HIV screening programmes, Geneva, 20–21 May 1987, WHO/SPA/GLO/87.2.

World Health Organization. (1987d) *Report of the consultation on international travel and HIV infection: Excerpts*. Geneva, 2–3 March 1987, WHO/SPA/GLO/87.1.

World Health Organization. (1987e) *Statement from the consultation on prevention and control of AIDS in prisons.* Geneva, 16–18 November 1987, WHO/SPA/INF/87.14.

World Health Organization. (1987f) *Report of the consultation on international travel and HIV infection.* (Excerpts) Geneva, 2–3 March 1987. WHO/SPA/GLO/87.1.

World Health Organization. (1987g) AIDS and the use of barrier methods, particularly condoms and spermicides. In: *Barrier Contraceptives and Spermicides.* Geneva, 1987.

World Health Organization. (1987h) *Note Verbale from the Director-General on the Prevention of HIV Transmission Through Skin Piercing Procedures.* 17 September 1987. C.L.30.

World Health Organization. (1987i) *Blood, Blood Products.* Report by the Director-General, Executive Board document EB/79/7 Add. (Geneva 1987).

World Health Organization. (1987j) Special Programme on AIDS Statement. *HIV Infection and Health Care Workers.* Washington, DC. 6 June 1987, SPA/INF/87.6.

World Health Organization. (1988a) Global Programme on AIDS. *Guiding Objectives and Principles for the Comprehensive Coordination of Global and National AIDS Activities.* Fifth Meeting of Participating Parties, Geneva, 27–28 April 1988, GPA/ER/88.2 Rev. 1.

World Health Organization. (1988b) *AIDS: Discrimination and public health* by Dr. Jonathan Mann, Director GPA/WHO, IV International Conference on AIDS, Stockholm, 13 June 1988.

World Health Organization. (1988c) *Report of the meeting on HIV infection and drug injecting intervention strategies: Recommendations.* WHO/GPA/SBR/89.1, Geneva, January 1988.

World Health Organization. (1988d) *Screening and testing in AIDS prevention and control programmes.* Geneva, January 1988, WHO/SPA/INF/88.1.

World Health Organization. (1988e) *Statement on screening of international travellers for infection with human immunodeficiency virus.* Geneva, 1988, WHO/GPA/INF/88.3.

World Health Organization. (1988f) *Consensus statement from the consultation on AIDS and the workplace.* Geneva, 27–29 June 1988. WHO/GPA/INF/88.7.

World Health Organization. (1988g) *Statement on screening of international travellers for infection with human immunodeficiency virus.* Geneva, 1988. WHO/GPA/INF/88.3.

World Health Organization. (1988h) *Report of the Global Blood Safety Initiative Meeting: Excerpts,* Geneva, 16–17 May 1988. WHO/GPA/DIR 88.9.

World Health Organization. (1989a) *Attention to Applicable International Law.* Recommendation 19 of the Global Commission on AIDS, Geneva, 29–31 March 1989, GPA/GCA(1)/89.1.

World Health Organization. (1989b) Statement by WHO collaborating centres on AIDS: *Heterosexual transmission of HIV and certain common social situations.* Geneva, January 1989, WHO/GPA/INF/89.5.

World Health Organization. (1989c) *Consensus statement from the consultation on sexually transmitted diseases as a risk factor for HIV transmission,* Geneva, 4–6 January 1989, WHO/.GPA/INF/89.1.

World Health Organization. (1989d) *Consensus statement from the consultation on partner notification for preventing HIV transmission: Excerpts.* Geneva, January 1989 WHO/GPA/INF/89.

World Health Organization. (1989e) *Consensus statement from the consultation on HIV epidemiology and prostitution,* Geneva, 3–6 July, 1989 WHO/GPA/INF/89.11.

World Health Organization. (1989f) *Unlinked anonymous screening for the public health surveillance of HIV infections. Proposed international guidelines,* Geneva, June 1989, GPA/SFI/89.3.

World Health Organization. (1989g) *Final Document: AIDS and Human Rights,* International Consultation on AIDS and Human Rights, Geneva, 26–28 July 1989, HR/AIDS/1989/3.

World Health Organization. (1989h,j) *Consensus Statement on Criteria for International Testing of Candidate Vaccines*; Excerpts, Geneva, 27 February–2 March 1989. GPA/INF/89.8.

World Health Organization. (1989i) Global Programme on AIDS. *Guidelines for Treatment of Acute Blood Loss*. Geneva. WHO/GPA/INF/88.5.

World Health Organization. (1990) *AIDS and Human Rights*, Report of a Regional Conference. Brazzaville, 12–16 March 1990.

World Health Organization. (1990a) *Consensus Statement from the Consultation on Global Strategies for Coordination of AIDS and STD Control Programmes*. Global Programme on AIDS and Programme of STD. Geneva, 11–13 July 1990. WHO/GPA/INF/90.2.

World Health Organization. (1991) Global Programme on AIDS. *Pan European Consultation on HIV/AIDS in the Context of Public Health and Human Rights*. Prague, 26–27 November 1991.

World Health Organization. (1991a) Global Programme on AIDS. *Country Watch: AIDS Health Promotion Exchange*. 2(1991):12.

World Health Organization. (1991b) Global Programme on AIDS. *Report of a WHO consultation on the prevention of human immunodeficiency virus and hepatitis B virus transmission in the health care setting*. Geneva, 11–12 April 1991. WHO/GPA/DIR/91.5.

World Health Organization. (1992) *Recommendations on Selection and Use of HIV Tests*. Geneva, May, 1992.

World Health Organization. (1992a) Global Programme on AIDS. *The Current Global Situation of the HIV/AIDS Pandemic*, July, 1992.

World Health Organization. (1992b) Global Programme on AIDS. *World AIDS Cases Quarterly Update*, 1 July 1992.

World Health Organization. (1992c) Global Programme on AIDS. *Tabular Information on Legal Instruments Dealing with HIV infection and AIDS*. Compiled by Sev Fluss. WHO/GPA/HLE/92.1, 9 June 1992.

World Health Organization. (1992d) *International Travel and Health: Vaccination and Health Advice*. Geneva, 1992.

World Health Organization. (1992e) *Tuberculosis Notification Update*. Tuberculosis Programme, Division of Communicable Diseases, WHO. Geneva, July 1992. WHO/TB/92.169.

World Health Organization. (1992f) *The Role of Sexually Transmitted Diseases in the Prevention and Control of AIDS*. Programme of Sexually Transmitted diseases (GPA/VDT). Geneva, 1992. WHO/VDT/INT/92.1.

World Health Organization. (1992g) *Effective Approaches to AIDS Prevention*. Conclusion of a meeting, May 26–29, 1992.

World Health Organization. (1992h) Global Programme on AIDS. *Statement from the Consultation on Testing and Counseling for HIV Infection*. Geneva, 16–18 November 1992.

World Health Organization. (1993) Global Programme on AIDS. *The HIV/AIDS Pandemic: 1993 Overview*. (1993). WHO/GPA/CNP/EVA/93.1.

World Health Organization. (1993a) Global Programme on AIDS. *Tabular Information on Legal Instruments Dealing with HIV Infection and AIDS*. Compiled by Sev Fluss. WHO/GPA/HLE/93.1.

World Health Organization. (1993b) Global Programme on AIDS. *Guidelines on HIV Infection and AIDS in Prisons*. Geneva, March 1993. WHO/GPA/DIR/93.3.

World Health Organization/United Nations International Children's Educational Fund (WHO/UNICEF). (1992) Statement on breast-feeding and HIV. WHO/UNICEF consultative meeting of April 30–May 1. *Weekly Epidemiological Review*. 67:177–184.

World Summit of Ministers of Health. (1988) *London declaration on AIDS prevention*. World Summit of Ministers of Health on programmes for AIDS prevention, London, 28 January 1988.

BOOKS AND BOOK-LENGTH MANUSCRIPTS

Allen AL. (1987) *Uneasy Access: Privacy for Women in a Free Society.* Totowa, NJ: Rowman & Littlefield.

Ankrah EM, Gostin LO. (1994) Ethical and Legal Considerations of the HIV Epidemic in Africa. In: Essex M, Mboup S, Kanki PJ, Kalengayi M (eds.) *AIDS in Africa.* New York: Raven Press.

Auerbach JD, Wypijewska C, Brodie HKH (eds.). (1994) *AIDS and Behavior.* Report of the Committee on Substance Abuse and Mental Health Issues in AIDS Research and Division of Biobehavioral Sciences and Mental Disorders, Institute of Medicine. Washington, DC: National Academy Press.

Bayer R. (1991) *Private Acts, Social Consequences: AIDS and the Politics of Public Health.* New Brunswick, NJ: Rutgers University Press.

Beal R, Britten AFH, Gust I. (1992) Blood Safety and Blood Products. In: Mann J, Tarantola DJM, Netter TW (eds.) *AIDS in the World 1992.* Cambridge, MA: Harvard University Press, pp. 421–437.

Beauchamp TL, Childress JF. (1994) *Principles of Biomedical Ethics, fourth edition.* New York, NY: Oxford University Press.

Bilder RB. (1986) An Overview of International Human Rights Law. In: Hannum H. (ed.) for the International Human Rights Law Group. *Guide to International Human Rights Practice.* Philadelphia, PA: University of Pennsylvania Press.

Brandt AM. (1987) *No Magic Bullet: A Social History of Venereal Disease in the United States Since 1880.* New York, NY: Oxford University Press.

Brandt AM, Cleary PD, Gostin LO. (1990) Routine Hospital Testing for HIV: Health Policy Considerations. In: Gostin LO (ed.) *AIDS and the Health Care System.* New Haven, CT: Yale University Press.

Britten AFH. (1988) *Role of the League of Red Cross and Red Crescent Societies,* Geneva, 1988. WHO doc. GBS/GPA/ISE.

Cassese A. (1990) *Human Rights in a Changing World.* Cambridge, MA: Polity.

Centers for Disease Control. (1994) *Addressing Emerging Infectious Disease Threats: A Prevention Strategy for the United States.* Atlanta, GA: National Center for Infectious Diseases (NCID), Public Health Service, U.S. Department of Health and Human Services.

Chapman AR. (1993) *Exploring a Human Rights Approach to Health Care Reform.* Washington, DC: American Association for the Advancement of Science.

Cohen R, Weisberg LS. (1990) *Double Jeopardy—Threat to Life and Human Rights.* Cambridge, MA: Human Rights Internet, March 1990.

Curran W, Gostin LO, Lazzarini Z. (1991) *International Survey of Legislation Relating to the AIDS Epidemic.* World Health Organization, Geneva (in publication).

Daniels N. (1985) *Just Health Care.* New York, NY: Cambridge University Press.

Daniels N. (1995) *Seeking Fair Treatment: From the AIDS Epidemic to National Health Care Reform.* New York, NY: Oxford University Press.

Dickens BM, Howe EG, Carroll AJ, Dreher D. (1992) HIV Screening: The International Implications. In: Gostin LO, Porter L (eds.) *International Law and AIDS.* Chicago, IL: American Bar Association, Section of International Law and Practice.

Diemer A. (1986) The 1948 Declaration: An Analysis of Meanings. In: *Philosophical foundations of human rights.* Prepared by UNESCO and the International Institute of Philosophy. Paris: United Nations Educational, Scientific and Cultural Organization.

Donnelly J. (1985) *The Concept of Human Rights.* New York, NY: St. Martin's Press.

Dorkenoo E, Elworthy S. (1992) *Female Genital Mutilation: Proposals for Change.* London, England: Minority Rights Group.

Drzemczewski A. (1983) *European Human Rights Convention in Domestic Law.*

Elias CJ, Heise L. (1993) *The Development of Microbicides: A New Method of HIV Prevention for Women.* New York, NY: Population Council. Working Paper Number 6.

Fuenzzlida-Puelma HL, Connor SS (eds.). (1989) *The Right to Health in the Americas: A Comparative Constitutional Study.* Washington, DC: Pan American Health Organization.

Gostin LO, Lazzarini Z. (1994) *Tuberculosis, the Law, and Public Health.* Agency for Health Care Policy and Research, United States Public Health Service.

Gostin LO, Lazzarini Z, Flaherty KM, Scherer R, Smith M. (1996) *The AIDS Litigation Project III: A Look at AIDS in the Courts in the 90s.* Menlo Park, CA: Kaiser Family Foundation.

Hammett TM. (1987) *AIDS in Correctional Facilities: Issues and Options. 2d ed. with 1986 update.* Washington, DC: National Institute of Justice.

Hammett TM. (1989) *AIDS in Correctional Facilities: Issues and Options. 2d ed. with 1988 update.* Washington, DC: National Institute of Justice.

Hannum H (ed). (1986) *Guide to International Human Rights Practice.* Philadelphia, PA: University of Pennsylvania Press.

Harvard Law School Human Rights Program. (1995) *Economic and Social Rights and the Right to Health: An Interdisciplinary Discussion Held at Harvard Law School in September, 1993.* Cambridge, MA: HRP.

Helie-Lucas MA. (1993) Women Living Under Muslim Laws. In: Kerr J (ed.) *Ours By Right: Women's Rights as Human Rights.* London and Ottawa: Zed Books and The North-South Institute, pp. 52–64.

Henkin L. (1979) *How Nations Behave.* New York, NY: Columbia University Press, p. 320.

Henkin L. (1990) *The Age of Rights.* New York, NY: Columbia University Press, p. 1.

Higgins R. (1994) *Problems and Process: International Law and How We Use It.* New York, NY: Oxford University Press, p. 99.

Human Rights Watch. (1995) *Human Rights Watch World Report 1995: Events of 1994.* New York, NY: Human Rights Watch.

Institute of Medicine. (1988) *The Future of Public Health.* Washington, DC: National Academy Press.

Institute of Medicine. (1992) *Emerging Infections: Microbial Threats to Health in the United States.* Lederberg J, Shope RE, Oaks SC (eds.) Washington, DC: National Academy Press.

Institute of Medicine. (1994) *AIDS and Behavior: An Integrated Approach.* Washington, DC: National Academy Press.

International Commission of Jurists. (1983) *States of Emergency: Their Impact on Human Rights.* Geneva: ICJ.

International Federation of Red Cross and Red Crescent Societies and François-Xavier Bagnoud Center for Health and Human Rights, Harvard School of Public Health (IFRC, FXB). (1995) *AIDS, Health and Human Rights: An explanatory manual.* Geneva and Boston, MA: International Federation of Red Cross and Red Crescent Societies and Harvard School of Public Health.

Levine RJ. (1982) Validity of Consent Procedures in Technologically Developing Countries. In: Bankowski Z, Howard-Jones J (eds.) *Human Experimentation and Medical Ethics.* Geneva: CIOMS, pp. 16–30.

Mann JM, Tarantola DJM, Netter TW (eds.). (1992) The HIV Pandemic: Status and Trends. In: *AIDS in the World 1992.* Cambridge, MA: Harvard University Press, pp. 11–108.

Mollica RF, Donelan K, Tor S, La Velle J, Elias C, Frankel M, Bennett D, Bundon RJ. (1991) *Repatriation and Disability: A Community Study of Health, Mental Health and Social Functioning of the Khmer Residents of Site 2.* Report sponsored by the World Federation for Mental Health. Baltimore, MD: Harvard School of Public Health, Boston, MA.

Normand J, Vlahov D, Moses LE (eds.). (1995) *Preventing HIV Transmission: The Role of Sterile Needles and Bleach.* Report of an expert panel convened by the National Research Council and Institute of Medicine. Washington, DC: National Academy Press.

Oraá J. (1992) *Human Rights in States of Emergency in International Law.* New York, NY: Oxford University Press.

Ozar DT. (1985) Rights: What They Are and Where They Come From. In: Werhane H, Gini AR, Ozar DT (eds.) *Philosophical Issues in Human rights Theories and Applications.* New York, NY: Random House.

Porter L, Gostin LO. (1992) *Legal Environment Surrounding the Availability of Sterile Needles and Syringes to Injecting Drug Users.* Report submitted jointly to the World Health Organization and the International Narcotics Control Board. United Nations.

Preston A, Armsby T. (1990) *What Works? Safer Injecting Guide.* Exeter, Devon: The Exeter Drugs Project.

Prevention of Maternal Mortality Network. (1990) *Barriers to Treatment of Obstetric Emergencies in West Africa: A Report of Focus Group Research in Nigeria, Ghana and Sierra Leone.* Background paper for the Safe Motherhood Conference, Abja, Nigeria, 11–13 September 1990.

Robertson AH, Merrills JG. (1989) *Human Rights in the World, Third Edition.* Manchester: Manchester University Press.

Sabatier R. (1988) *Blaming Others: Prejudice, Race and World-Wide AIDS.* London, England: Panos Institute.

San Francisco AIDS Foundation. (1989) Transmission of HIV Among Intravenous Drug Users. In: Hellman S, Rosenberg SA (eds.) *AIDS: Etiology, Diagnosis, Treatment and Prevention.* 385 VT DeVita.

Schachter O. (1991) *International Law in Theory and Practice.* Nordrecht, The Netherlands: M. Nijhoff Publishers.

Sen G, Germain A, Chen LC (eds.) (1994) *Population Policies Reconsidered.* Boston, MA: Harvard Series on Population and International Health, Harvard Center for Population and Development Studies, distributed by Harvard University Press.

Sen G, Snow R (eds.). (1994) *Power and Decision: The Social Control of Reproduction.* Boston, MA: Harvard Series on Population and International Health, Harvard Center for Population and Development Studies, distributed by Harvard University Press.

Shelton DL. (1986) Individual Complaint Machinery Under the United Nations 1503 Procedure and the Optional Protocol to the International Covenant on Civil and Political Rights. In: Hannum H (ed.) for the International Human Rights Law Group. *Guide to International Human Rights Practice.* Philadelphia, PA: University of Pennsylvania Press.

Shestack J. (1978) Sisyphus Endures: The International Human Rights NGO. 24 *New York School of Law Review* 89.

Shue H. (1979) Rights in the Light of Duties. In: Brown PG, MacLean D (eds.) *Human rights and U.S. Foreign Policy.* Lexington, MA: Lexington Books.

Shue H. (1980) *Basic Rights.* Princeton, NJ: Princeton University Press.

Sieghart P. (1985) *The Lawful Rights of Mankind: An Introduction to the International Legal Code of Human Rights.* Oxford, New York, NY: Oxford University Press.

Steiner H. (1991) *Diverse Partners: Non-Governmental Organizations in the Human Rights Movement.* Report of a meeting in Crete 1989.

Stryker J, Samuels SE, Smith MD. (1993) Executive Summary. In: Samuels SE, Smith MD (eds.) *Condoms in the Schools.* Menlo Park, CA: Kaiser Family Foundation.

Stryker J, Smith MD (eds.). (1993) *Dimensions of HIV Prevention: Needle Exchange.* Menlo Park, CA: Henry J. Kaiser Family Foundation.

Tomasevski K, Gruskin S, Lazzarini Z, Hendriks A. (1992) AIDS and Human Rights. In: Mann J, Tarantola DJM, Netter TW (eds.) *AIDS in the World 1992*. Cambridge, MA: Harvard University Press, pp. 537–573.

Tomasevski K. (1994) *Human Rights in Population Policies*. Lund, Sweden: SIDA.

United Nations Yearbook. (1948) Lake Success, NY: U.N.

Widdows K. (1993) International Labor Law and AIDS. In: Gostin LG, Porter L (eds.) *AIDS and International Law: International Responses, Current Issues, and Future Directions*. Chicago, IL: American Bar Association.

ARTICLES

Adityanjee D. (1986) Informed consent: issues involved for developing countries. *Medicine, Science and Law* 26:305–307.

Ajayi OO. (1980) Taboos and clinical research in West Africa. *Journal of Medical Ethics* 1980:6061–6063.

Altman LK. (1994) In major finding, drug curbs HIV infection in newborns. *New York Times*. February 21, 1994; A1.

Alston P. (1993a) Democracy, development and human tights. Paper presented at: Interregional meeting organized by the Council of Europe in advance of the World Conference on Human Rights, entitled *Human Rights at the Dawn of the 21st Century*. Palais del'Europe, Strasbourg, 28–30 January 1993. Strasbourg: Council of Europe Press.

American Medical Association. (1995) Female genital mutilation: report of the council on scientific affairs. *Journal of the American Medical Association* 274:1714–1720.

Amnesty International. (1984) *Torture in the Eighties*. London, England: Amnesty International.

Amnesty International. (1993) *Amnesty International Report 1993*. London, England: Amnesty International.

Andrus JK, Fleming DW, Knox C, McAlister RO, Skeels MR, Conrad RE, Horan JM, Foster LR. (1989) HIV testing in prisoners: is mandatory testing mandatory? *American Journal of Public Health* 79:840–842.

Arno PS, Murray CJL, Bonuck KA, Alcabes P. (1993) The economic impact of tuberculosis in New York city: a preliminary analysis. *Journal of Law, Medicine and Ethics* 21:317–323.

Bardsley J, Turvey J, Blatherwick J. (1990) Vancouver's needle exchange program. *Canadian Journal of Public Health* 81:39–45.

Bauder D. (1994) Secrecy law under fire for hiding baby's AIDS infection from mother; health: a New York legislative proposal to "unblind" neonatal tests has become the subject of a fierce fight. The debate transcends political lines and even divides doctors who treat the disease. *Los Angeles Times*. April 17; A8.

Basoglu M, Paker M, Ozmen E, Tasdemir O, Sahin D. (1994) Factors related to long-term traumatic stress responses in survivors of torture in Turkey. *Journal of the American Medical Association* 272(5):357–363.

Bayer R. (1991) Public health policy and the AIDS epidemic: an end to HIV exceptionalism? *New England Journal of Medicine* 324:1500–1504.

Bayer R. (1994) Ethical challenges posed by zidovudine treatment to reduce vertical transmission of HIV. *New England Journal of Medicine* 318:1223–1225.

Bayer R. (1995) It's not 'Tuskegee' revisited: the false furor over HIV testing and newborn babies. *New York Times*. May 26; A27.

Bayer R, Healton C. (1989) Controlling AIDS in Cuba: the logic of quarantine. *New England Journal of Medicine* 320:1022.

Bayer R, Lumey LH, Wan L. (1991) The American, British and Dutch response to unlinked anonymous HIV seroprevalence studies: an international comparison. *Law, Medicine and Health Care* 19:222–230.

Becker MH, Joseph JG. (1988) AIDS and behavioral change to reduce risk: a review. *American Journal of Public Health* 78:394–410.

Bryson Y. (1996) *Perinatal transmission: associated factors and therapeutic approaches.* Plenary address at the XI International Conference on AIDS, Vancouver, Canada, 7–12 July 1996.

Burris S. (1992) HIV education and the law: a critical review. *Law, Medicine and Health Care* 20:377–391.

Burris S. (1994) Public health, "AIDS exceptionalism" and the law. *John Marshall Law Review* 27:251–272.

Caldwell MB, Fleming PL, Oxtoby MJ. (1992) Estimated number of AIDS orphans in the United States. *Pediatrics* 90:482.

Capron A. (1989) Protection of research subjects: do special rules apply in epidemiology? Paper presented the IEF Conference on Ethics in Epidemiology, Birmingham, Alabama, 12–13 June 1989.

Centers for Disease Control and Prevention. (1981) Kaposi's sarcoma and pneumocystis pneumonia among homosexual men—New York City and California. *Morbidity and Mortality Weekly Report* 30:305–308.

Centers for Disease Control and Prevention. (1987) Public health service guidelines for counseling and anti-body testing to prevent HIV infection and AIDS. *Morbidity and Mortality Weekly Report* 36(31):509–515.

Centers for Disease Control and Prevention. (1990) *HIV/AIDS surveillance: U.S. cases reported through September.*

Centers for Disease Control and Prevention. (1990a) Guidelines for preventing the transmission of tuberculosis in health-care settings, with special focus on HIV-related issues. *Morbidity and Mortality Weekly Report* 39 (RR-17).

Centers for Disease Control and Prevention. (1991) Tuberculosis outbreak among persons in a residential facility for HIV-infected persons—San Francisco. *Morbidity and Mortality Weekly Report* 40:649–652.

Centers for Disease Control and Prevention. (1991a) Recommendations for preventing transmission of human immunodeficiency virus and hepatitis B virus to patients during exposure-prone invasive procedures. *Morbidity and Mortality Weekly Report* 40 (No. RR-8):1–6.

Centers for Disease Control and Prevention. (1993) Update: investigations of persons treated by HIV-infected health care workers-United States. *Morbidity and Mortality Weekly Report* 42:329–332.

Centers for Disease Control and Prevention. (1993a) Quantification of HIV-1 transmission risk associated with breastfeeding: the case for randomized infant feeding trials. Case developed by Nieburg P, DeCock KM, Oxtoby M. Division of HIV/AIDS; project RETRO-CI, Abidjan, Cote d'Ivoire.

Centers for Disease Control and Prevention. (1993b) Recommendations for HIV testing services for inpatients in acute-care hospital settings. *Morbidity and Mortality Weekly Report* 42 (No. RR-2):1–17.

Centers for Disease Control and Prevention. (1994) Zidovudine for the prevention of HIV transmission from mother to infant. *Morbidity and Mortality Weekly Report* 43(16):285–287.

Centers for Disease Control and Prevention. (1994a) Surveillance of health care workers exposed to blood from HIV-positive patients. CDC Fax Information Service, Document # 370159, 15 September.

Centers for Disease Control and Prevention. (1994b) Guidelines for preventing the transmission of *Mycobacterium tuberculosis* in health-care facilities, 1994. *Morbidity and Mortality Weekly Report* 43 (No. RR-13):1–132.

Centers for Disease Control and Prevention. (1995a) 1995 Revised guidelines for prophylaxis against Pneumocystis carinii pneumonia for children infected with or perinatally exposed to human immunodeficiency virus. *Morbidity and Mortality Weekly Report* 44 (No. RR-4):1–11.

Centers for Disease Control and Prevention. (1995b) USPHS/IDSA guidelines for the prevention of opportunistic infections in persons infected with human immunodeficiency virus: a summary. *Morbidity and Mortality Weekly Report* 44 (No. RR-8):1–34.

Centers for Disease Control and Prevention. (1995c) U.S. Public Health Service recommendations for human immunodeficiency virus counseling and voluntary testing for pregnant women. *Morbidity and Mortality Weekly Report* 44 (No. RR-7):1–15.

Centers for Disease Control and Prevention. (1995d) Syringe exchange programs—United States, 1994–1995. *Morbidity and Mortality Weekly Report* 44:684–685, 691.

Centers for Disease Control and Prevention. (1995e) *HIV/AIDS surveillance report, 1994.* Atlanta, Georgia: U.S. Department of Health and Human Services, Public Health Service 6:11–12.

Centers for Disease Control and Prevention. (1995f) Essential components of a tuberculosis prevention and control program; and screening for tuberculosis and tuberculosis infection in high-risk populations: recommendations of the advisory council for the elimination of tuberculosis. *Morbidity and Mortality Weekly Report* 44 (No. RR-11):1–34.

Centers for Disease Control and Prevention. (1995g) Case-control study of HIV seroconversion in health-care workers after percutaneous exposure to HIV-infected blood—France, United Kingdom, and United States, January 1988–August 1994. *Morbidity and Mortality Weekly Report* 44:929–933.

Centers for Disease Control and Prevention. (1996) Identification of HIV-1 group O infection—Los Angeles County, California, 1996. *Morbidity and Mortality Weekly Report* 45:561–565.

Centers for Disease Control and Prevention. (1996a) Update: provisional public health service recommendations for chemoprophylaxis after occupational exposure to HIV. *Morbidity and Mortality Weekly Report* 45:468–472.

Chambuso SA. (1991) AIDS in prison: the Tanzanian experience. Presented at a seminar on prison medicine. International Committee of the Red Cross, Port Louis, Mauritius.

Chen LH, Souza SA. (1981) Sex bias in the family allocation of food and health care in rural Bangladesh. *Population and Development Review* March 1981.

Choopanya K, Vanichiseni S, Des Jarlais DC. (1991) Risk factors and HIV seropositivity among injecting drug users in Bangkok. *Journal of Acquired Immune Deficiency Syndrome* 5:1509–1513.

Christakis NA. (1988) The ethical design of an AIDS vaccine trial in Africa. *Hastings Center Report* 18:31–37.

Christakis NA. (1989) Responding to a pandemic: international interests in AIDS control. *Daedalus* 118:113–134.

Cleary PD, Barry MJ, Mayer KH, Brandt AM, Gostin LO, Fineberg HV. (1987) Compulsory premarital screening for the human immunodeficiency-virus. *Journal of the American Medical Association* 258:1757–1762.

Cook RJ. (1992) International protection of women's reproductive rights. *New York University Journal of International Law & Politics* 24(2):645–772.

Cook RJ. (1993) International human rights and women's reproductive health. *Studies in Family Planning* 24(2):73–86.

D'Aquila, RT Williams, AB. (1987) Epidemic human immunodeficiency virus (HIV) infection among intravenous drug users. *Yale Journal of Biology and Medicine* 60:545–567.

Dalton H. (1989) AIDS in blackface. 118 *Daedalus* 205:222–224.

Dawit S, Mekuria S. (1993) The west just doesn't get it. *New York Times.* December 1993.

DeCock KM, Ekpini E, Gnaore E, Kadio A, Gayle HD. (1994) The public health implications o AIDS research in Africa. *Journal of the American Medical Association* 272:481–486.

DeCock KM, Soro B, Coulibaly IM, Lucas SB. (1992) Tuberculosis and HIV infection in Sub Saharan Africa. *Journal of the American Medical Association* 268:1581–1587.

DeJong W. (1989) Condom promotion: the need for a social marketing program in America' inner cities. *American Journal of Health Promotion* 3:5–16.

Des Jarlais D, Friedman SR. (1988) The psychology of preventing AIDS among intravenou drug users. *American Psychologist* 43:865.

De Vincenzi I. (1994) European study group on heterosexual transmission of HIV. A longitudi nal study of human immunodeficiency virus transmission by heterosexual partners. *Nev England Journal of Medicine* 331:341–346.

Donoghoe MC, Stimson GV, Dolan K, Alldritt L. (1989) Changes in HIV risk behavior in cli ents of syringe-exchange schemes in England and Scotland. *Journal of Acquired Immun Deficiency Syndrome* 3:267–272.

Duckett M, Orkin AJ. (1989) AIDS-related migration and travel policies and restrictions: a glo bal survey. *AIDS* 3(Suppl. 1):S231–252 A Year in Review, Current Science, Philadelphia.

Dunn DT, Newell ML, Ades AE, Peckham CS. (1992) Risk of human immunodeficiency type transmission through breastfeeding. *Lancet* 340:585–588.

The Economist. (1993) The blue and the red. *The Economist.* 8 May 1993, pp. 19–20.

Edgar H, Sandomire H. (1989) Medical privacy issues in the age of AIDS: legislative options *American Journal of Law and Medicine* 76(1–2):155–210.

Ekunwe EO, Kessel R. (1984) Informed consent in the developing world. *Hastings Center Re port* 14:23–24.

European Collaborative Study. (1992) Risk factors for mother-to-child transmission of HIV-1 *Lancet* 339:1007–1012.

Field M. (1990) Testing for AIDS: uses and abuses. *American Journal of Law and Medicin* 16:33–106.

Fischl MA, Richman PD, Grieco MH. (1987) The efficacy of azidothymidine (AZT) in treatmen of AIDS and AIDS-related complex. *New England Journal of Medicine* 317:185–191.

Francis DP, Curran JW, Essex M. (1983) Epidemic acquired immune deficiency syndrome: epi demiological evidence for a transmissible agent. *Journal of the National Cancer Institut* 71:1–4.

Freudenberg N. (1990) AIDS prevention in the United States: Lessons from the first decade *International Health Services* 20:590–598.

Frieden TR, Fujiwara PI, Washko RM, Hamburg MA. (1995) Tuberculosis in New York City— turning the tide. *New England Journal of Medicine* 333:229–233.

Garrett L, Woodward C. (1992) TB in NY: new risk in hospitals: study shows 19 workers con tract TB. *New York Newsday.* March 10, 1992, pp. 6, 26.

Geiger JH, Cook-Deegan RM. (1993) The role of physicians in conflicts and humanitarian cri ses. *Journal of the American Medical Association* 270:616–620.

Gostin LO, Cleary PD, Mayer KH, Brandt AM, Chittendon EH. (1990) Screening immigrant and international travelers for the human immunodeficiency virus. *New England Journal o Medicine* 322:1743–1746.

Gostin LO. (1986) The future of public health law. *American Journal of Law and Medicin* 12:461–490.

Gostin LO. (1989) Public health strategies for controlling AIDS: legislation and regulatory policy in the United States. *Journal of the American Medical Association* 261(11):1621–1630.

Gostin LO. (1990a) The AIDS litigation project: a national review of court and human rights commission decisions. Part I: The social impact of AIDS. *Journal of the American Medical Association* 263(14):1961–1970.

Gostin LO. (1990b) The AIDS litigation project: a national review of court and human rights commission decisions. Part II: discrimination. *Journal of the American Medical Association* 263(15):2086–2092.

Gostin LO. (1991) Ethical principles for the conduct of human subject research: population-based research and ethics. *Law, Medicine and Health Care* 19:3, 4, 191.

Gostin LO. (1991b) The interconnected epidemics of drug dependency and AIDS. *Harvard Civil Rights Civil Liberties Law Review* 26(1):113–184.

Gostin LO. (1992a) Human Rights for Persons with Mental Illness: An International Approach Based Upon the European Convention of Human Rights. To appear in: Polubinskya S, Shah SA (eds.) *Law, Mental Health and Human Rights: Russian and American Perspectives.* (in press).

Gostin LO. (1993) Law and Policy. In: Stryker J, Smith MD (eds.) *Dimensions of HIV Prevention: Needle Exchange.* Menlo Park, CA: Henry J. Kaiser Family Foundation, pp. 35–62.

Gostin LO, Mann J. (1994) Towards the development of a human rights impact assessment for the formulation and evaluation of health policies. *Health and Human Rights An International Quarterly Journal* 1:58–81.

Gostin LO. (1995) The resurgent tuberculosis epidemic in the era of AIDS: reflections on public health, law, and society. *Maryland Law Review* 54:1–131.

Gostin LO. (1995b). Health information privacy. *Cornell Law Review* 80:101–184.

Gostin LO, Lazzarini Z, Neslund VS, Osterholm MT. (1996a) The public health information infrastructure: a national review of health information privacy. *Journal of the American Medical Association* 275:1921–1927.

Gostin LO, Lazzarini Z, Flaherty KM, Jones TS. (1996b) *Limitations on the sale and possession of syringes; results of a national survey of laws and regulations.* Report, unpublished, to the Centers for Disease Control and Prevention.

Greenhouse L. (1993) High court backs policy of halting Haitian refugees. *New York Times.* June 22, 1993, pp. A1, A18.

Groseclose SL, Weinstein B, Jones TS. (1995) Impact of increased legal access to needles and syringes on practices of injecting drug users and police officers—Connecticut, 1992–1993. *Journal of Acquired Immune Deficiency Syndrome* 10:82–89.

Gruskin S. (1995) Women's health and human rights. Special issue of *Health and Human Rights: An International Journal* 1 (4):309–497.

Hagan H, Des Jarlais DC, Purchase D, Reid T, Friedman SR. (1991) The Tacoma syringe exchange. *Journal of Addictive Diseases* 10 (4):81–88.

Hall AJ. (1989) Public health trials in West Africa: logistics and ethics. *IRB* 11:8.

Halsey NA, Boulos R, Holt E, Ruff A, Brutus J-R, Kissinger P, Quinn TC, Coberly JS, Adrien M, Boulos C. (1990) Transmission of HIV-1 infections from mothers to infants in Haiti. *Journal of the American Medical Association* 264:2088–2092.

Hamblin J, Reid E. (1991) "Women, the HIV epidemic and human rights: a tragic imperative," paper presented to the Global Expert Meeting: AIDS, a Question of Rights and Humanity, The Hague. 21–24 May 1991.

Hammer SM. (1996) *Advances in antiretroviral therapy and viral load monitoring.* Plenary address at the XI International Conference on AIDS, Vancouver, Canada, 7–12 July 1996.

Hanson K. (1992) *The economic impact of AIDS: an assessment of the available evidence,* report commissioned by the Global Programme on AIDS, World Health Organization. 1 March 1992.

Harding TW. (1987) AIDS in prison. *Lancet* 2:1260–1263.

Harding TW, Schaller G. (1992) HIV AIDS Policy for Prisons or for Prisoners? In: Mann J, Tarantola DJM, Netter TW (eds.) *AIDS in the World 1992.* Cambridge, MA: Harvard University Press, 761–769.

Hart GH, Carvell ALM, Woodward N, Johnson AM, Williams P, Parry JV. (1989) Evaluation of needle exchange in central London: behaviour change and anti-HIV status over one year. *Journal of Acquired Immune Deficiency Syndrome* 3:261–265.

Hartgers C, Buning EC, van Santen GV, Verster AD, Coutinho RA. (1989) The impact of needle and syringe-exchange programme in Amsterdam on injecting risk behaviour. *Journal of Acquired Immune Deficiency Syndrome* 3:571–576.

Harvard Study Team. (1991) The Effect of the Gulf crisis on the children of Iraq. *New England Journal of Medicine* 325:977–980, September 26, 1991.

Hausermann J, Danziger R. (1991) "Women and AIDS: a human rights perspective," paper presented by Rights and Humanity at the VIIth International conference on AIDS, Florence, June 1991.

Heimer R. (1994) Presentation at focus group on HIV and substance abuse, July 28, Washington, DC.

Hellinger FJ. (1993) The lifetime cost of treating a person with HIV. *Journal of the American Medical Association* 270:474–478.

Henderson RH, Davis H, Eddins DL, Forge WH. (1973) Assessment of vaccination coverage, vaccination scar rates and small pox scarring in five areas of West Africa. *Bulletin of the World Health Organization* 48:183–194.

Hendriks A. (1992) Living with HIV/AIDS: a room of one's own. In: Mann J, Tarantola DJM, Netter TW (eds.) *AIDS in the World 1992.* Cambridge, MA: Harvard University Press, 769–774.

Hendriks A, Leckie S. (1991) *AIDS and Housing Rights in Western Europe: A Comparative Study of the Netherlands, Spain and the United Kingdom.* London: The National AIDS Trust.

Heymann DL, Bres P, Karam M, Biritvum R, Nkovane B, Sow A, Kenya P, Beausoleil EG, Widdus R, Mann JM. (1990) AIDS-related research in sub-Saharan Africa. *Journal of Acquired Immune Deficiency Syndrome* 4:469–470.

Heymann SJ. (1990) Modeling the impact of breast-feeding by HIV-infected women on child survival. *American Journal of Public Health* 80:1305–1309.

Higgins DL, Galavotti C, O'Reilly KR, Schnell DJ. (1991) Evidence for the effects of HIV antibody counseling and testing on risk behaviors. *Journal of the American Medical Association* 266:2419–2429.

Ho DD. (1996) *How long should treatment be given if we had an antiretroviral regimen that completely blocks HIV replication?* Abstract Th.B.930, presented at the XI International Conference on AIDS, Vancouver, Canada, 7–12 July 1996.

Hu DJ, Heyward WL, Byers RH, Nkowana BM, Oxtoby MJ, Holck SE, Heymann DL. (1992) HIV infection and breast-feeding: policy implications through a decision analysis model. *Journal of Acquired Immune Deficiency Syndrome* 6:1505–1512.

Hunter M. (1993) True horror: the french blood scandal. *Sacramento Bee.* 29 August 1993; F1.

Jallow H. (1991) *AIDS and human rights in the context of the African charter on human and peoples' rights,* paper presented to the Global Expert Meeting: AIDS, a Question of Rights and Humanity, The Hague, 21–24 May 1991, published as an occasional paper by the African Centre for Democracy and Human Rights Studies, Banjul, The Gambia.

Jamar SD. (1994) The international human right to health. *Southern University Law Review* 22:1–68.

Joseph SC, Des Jarlais DC. (1989) Needle and syringe exchange as a method of AIDS epidemic control. *AIDS Update* 2(5):1–8.

Kiragu J. (1995) HIV Prevention and women's rights: working for one means working for both. *AIDS Captions* Family Health International. November 1995; II(3):40–46.

Kirby D. (1993) Research and education. In: Samuels SE, Smith MD (eds.) *Condoms in the Schools*. Menlo Park, CA: Kaiser Family Foundation.

Kirby D, Waszak C, Ziegler J. (1991) Six school-based clinics: their reproductive health services and impact on sexual behavior. *Family Planning Perspectives* 23:6–16.

Klee H, Faugier J, Hayes C, Morris J. (1991) The sharing of injecting equipment among drug users attending prescribing clinics and those using needle-exchanges. *British Journal of Addiction* 86:217–223.

Kleinman S, Secord K. (1988) Risk of human immunodeficiency virus (HIV) transmission by anti-HIV negative blood. Estimates using the lookback methodology. *Transfusion* 28:499–501.

Koester SK. (1994) Copping, running, and paraphernalia laws: contextual variables and needle risk behavior among injection drug users in Denver. *Human Organization* Fall;53:287–295.

Koopman C, Rosario M, Rotheram-Borus MJ. (1994) Alcohol and drug use and sexual behaviors placing runaways at risk of HIV infection. *Addictive Behaviors* Jan-Feb;19:95–103.

Krauss C. (1993) Senate opposes immigration of people with AIDS virus. *New York Times*. 19 February 1993, p. A11.

Lackritz EM, Satten GA, Aberle-Grasse J, Dodd RY, Raimondi VP, Janssen RS, Lewis WF, Notari EP, IV, Petersen LR. (1995). Estimated risk of transmission of the human immunodeficiency virus by screened blood in the United States. *New England Journal of Medicine* 333:1721–1725.

Laga M, Nzila N, Goeman J. (1991) The interrelationship of sexually transmitted diseases and HIV infection: implications for the control of both epidemics in Africa. *AIDS* 5 (suppl. 1):S55–S63.

Lancet editorial. (1991) A European committee looks at degrading treatment. *Lancet* 338: 1559–1560.

Lalumiere C. (1993) Why this interregional meeting organized by the council of Europe? Opening Statement by the Secretary General of the Council of Europe at: Interregional meeting organized by the Council of Europe in advance of the World Conference on Human Rights, entitled *Human Rights at the Dawn of the 21st Century*. Palais del'Europe, Strasbourg, 28–30 January 1993. Strasbourg: Council of Europe Press.

Leary VA. (1994) The right to health in international human rights law. *International Journal of Health and Human Rights* 1:25–56.

Leckie S. (1990) "Access to Justice." In: *The Third Epidemic: Repercussions of the Fear of AIDS*. London, England: PANOS Institute, in association with the Norwegian Red Cross.

Leckie S. (1992) *From Housing Needs to Housing Rights: An Analysis of the Right to Housing Under International Human Rights Law*. London, England: International Institute for Environment and Development.

Lederman SA.(1992) Estimating infant mortality from human immunodeficiency virus and other causes in breast-feeding and bottle-feeding populations. *Pediatrics* 89:290–296.

Levine C. (1986) AIDS: Public health and civil liberties (Introduction). *Hastings Center Report* 16(1) (suppl December 1986).

Levine C, Dubler NN. (1990) HIV and childbearing: uncertain risks and bitter realities: the reproductive choices of HIV-infected women. *The Milbank Quarterly* 68(3):321–351.

Lichtenberg J. (1982) The moral equivalence of action and omission. *Canadian Journal of Philosophy* (suppl)8:19–36.

Liskin LS, Sakondhavat C. (1992) The Female Condom: A New Option for Women. In: Mann J, Tarantola DJM, Netter TW (eds.) *AIDS in the World 1992*. Cambridge, MA: Harvard University Press.

Ljungberg B, Christensson B, Tunving K, Andersson B, Landvall B, Lundberg M, Zall-Friberg A-C. (1991) HIV prevention among injecting drug users: three years of experience from a syringe exchange program in Sweden. *Journal of Acquired Immune Deficiency Syndrome* 4:890–895.

Lurie P, Reingold AL, Bowser D. (1993) *The Public Health Impact of Needle Exchange Programs in the United States and Abroad, Volume 1*. San Francisco, CA: University of California.

Macedo CG. (1988) Infant mortality in the Americas. *PAHO Bulletin* 22:303–312.

Mann JM, Gostin LO, Gruskin S, Brennan T, Lazzarini Z, Fineberg H. (1994) Health and human rights. *International Journal of Health and Human Rights* 1:7–23.

Marriott M. (1988) Needle exchange angers many minorities *New York Times*. November 7, 1988, p. 1, col. 2.

Masur H, Michelis MA, Greene JB, Onorato I, Stouve RA, Holzman RS, Wormser G, Brettman L, Lange M, Murray HW, Cunningham-Rundles S. (1981). An outbreak of community-acquired pneumocystis carinii pneumonia: initial manifestation of cellular immune dysfunction. *New England Journal of Medicine* 305:1431–1438.

Michaels D, Levine C. (1992) Estimates of the number of motherless youth orphaned by AIDS in the United States. *Journal of the American Medical Association* 268:3456–3461.

Minkoff H, Willoughby A. (1995) Pediatric disease, zidovudine in pregnancy, and unblinding heelstick surveys: reframing the debate on prenatal HIV testing. *Journal of the American Medical Association* 274:1165–1168.

Mollica RF, Caspi-Yavin Y. (1991) Measuring torture and torture-related symptoms. *Psychological Assessment* 3(4):1–7.

Mollica RF, Donelan K, Tor S, Lavelle J, Elias C, Frankel M, Blendon RJ. (1993) The effect of trauma and confinement on functional health and mental health status of Cambodians living in Thailand-Cambodia border camps. *Journal of the American Medical Association* 270: 581–586.

Moore RD, Stanton D, Goplan R, Chaisson RE. (1994) Racial differences in the use of drug therapy for HIV disease in an urban community. *The New England Journal of Medicine* 330:763–768.

National Institute on Drug Abuse—U.S. (1993) Community alert bulletin: proposed recommendations to prevent HIV transmission by sharing drug injection equipment, 23 March 1993.

Nelson KE, Vlahov D, Cohn S, Lindsay A, Solomon L, Anthony JC. (1991) Human immunodeficiency virus infection in diabetic intravenous drug users. *Journal of the American Medical Association* 266:2259–2261.

Neville K, Bromberg A, Bromberg R, Bonk S, Hanna BA, Rom WN. (1994) The third epidemic—multidrug-resistant tuberculosis. *Chest* January; 105:45–48.

New York City Department of Health. (1989) *The Pilot Exchange Study in New York City: A Bridge to Treatment* 4.

Nicoll A. (1993) International research on transmission of HIV-1 in relation to breast feeding: some notes from a public health perspective. Presented to the National Institutes of Health Workshop on Ethical Considerations in International Research on HIV Transmission Through Breastfeeding. 24 June 1993, Rockville, MD: NIH.

Nicoll A, Killewo JZJ, Mgone C. (1990) HIV and infant feeding practices: epidemiological implications for sub-Saharan African countries. *Journal of Acquired Immune Deficiency Syndrome* 4:661–665.

North RL, Rothenberg KH. (1993) Partner notification and the threat of domestic violence against women with HIV infection. *New England Journal of Medicine* 329:1194–1196.

N'tita I, Mulanga K, Dulat C, Lusamba D, Rehle H, Korbe R, Jager H. (1991) Risk of transfusion-associated HIV transmission in Kinshasa, Zaire. *Journal of Acquired Immune Deficiency Syndrome* 5(4)(1991): 437–439.

Padian NS, O'Brien TR, Chang YC, Glass S, Francis DP. (1993) Prevention of heterosexual transmission of human immunodeficiency virus through couple counseling. *Journal of Acquired Immune Deficiency Syndrome* 6:1043–1048.

Palasanthiran P, Ziegler JB, Stewart GJ, Stuckey M, Armstrong JA, Cooper DA, Penny R, Gold J. (1993) Breast-feeding during primary maternal human immunodeficiency virus infection and risk of transmission from mother to infant. *Journal of Infectious Diseases* February; 167:441–444.

Pantaleo G, Graziosi C, Fauci AS. (1993) The immunopathogenesis of human immunodeficiency virus infection. *New England Journal of Medicine* 328(5):327–334.

Paone D, Des Jarlais DC, Caloir S, Friedmann I. (1994) New York City syringe exchange: an overview. In *Proceedings, Workshop on Needle Exchange and Bleach Distribution Programs.* National Research Council and Institute of Medicine. Washington, DC: National Academy Press pp.47–63.

Pappas G, Queen S, Hadden W, Fisher G. (1993) The increasing disparity in mortality between socioeconomic groups in the United States, 1960 and 1986. *The New England Journal of Medicine* 329:103–109.

Parker R. (1996) *Empowerment, community mobilisation and social change in the face of HIV/ AIDS.* Plenary address at the XI International Conference on AIDS, Vancouver, Canada, 7–12 July 1996.

Picken M. (1985) *The role of the NGO in the implementation of human rights within the framework of the UN.* Paper delivered at University of Montreal Colloquium.

Pope John Paul II. (1989) Address of the Holy Father of the Fourth Intern. Conference promoted by the Pontifical Council for pastoral assistance to health care workers, the Vatican, 1989.

Porter K, Stryker J, Osborn J. (1992) HIV, AIDS and international travel. In: Gostin LO, Porter L (eds.) *International Law and AIDS.* Chicago, IL: American Bar Association.

Preble E. (1990) *Impact of HIV/AIDS on African children.* World Health Organization/UNICEF. March 1990.

Ravindran S. (1986) *Health implications of sex discrimination in childhood.* World Health Organization/UNICEF, FHE.86.2.

Reid E. (1990) *Placing women at the centre of the analyses.* Proceedings of the Meeting on Women and AIDS (forthcoming). Ottawa, Canada: CIDA. 1990.

Riding A. (1994) Scandal over tainted blood widens in France. *New York Times.* 13 February 1994, p. A16.

Ruff AJ, Halsey NA, Coberly J, Boulos R. (1992) Breast-feeding and maternal-infant transmission of human immunodeficiency virus type 1. *Journal of Pediatrics* 121:325–327.

Sande MA, Carpenter CCJ, Cobbs CG, Holmes KK, Sanford JP. (1993) Antiretroviral therapy for adult HIV-infected patients: recommendations from a state-of-the-art conference. *Journal of the American Medical Association* 270:2583–2589.

Sandler RH, Epstein PR, Cook-Deegan RM, Shukri A. (1991) Initial medical assessment of Kurdish refugees in the Turkey-Iraq border region. *Journal of the American Medical Association* 266:638–640.

Savand M-A. (1979) Why we are against the international campaign. *International Child Welfare Revue* 40:38.

Savarit D, DeCock KM, Schutz R, Konate S, Lackritz E, Bondurand A. (1992) Risk of HIV infection from transfusion with blood negative for HIV antibody in a West African city. *British Journal of Medicine* 305:498–502.

Schutz R, Savarit D, Kadjo J-C, Batter V, Kone N'V, La Ruche G, Bondurand A, DeCock KM. (1993) Excluding blood donors at high risk of HIV infection in a West African city. *British Medical Journal* 307:1517–1519.

Shreedhar J. (1995) Passage through India: HIV maps a deadly course. *Harvard AIDS Review* Fall:2–9.

Snider DE, Roper WL. (1992) The new tuberculosis. *The New England Journal of Medicine* 326:703–705.

San Francisco Chronicle. (1991) AIDS more prevalent among the homeless. (anonymous) San Francisco, CA, 18 June 1991.

Selwyn PA, Hartel D, Lewis VA, Schoenbaum EE, Vermund SH, Klein RS, Walker AT, Friedland GH. (1989) A prospective study of the risk of tuberculosis among intravenous drug users with human immunodeficiency virus infection. *New England Journal of Medicine* 320: 545–550.

Stimson GV, Hunter G, Rhodes T, Des Jarlais DC. (1996) *Continued global diffusion of injecting drug use has major implications for spread of HIV-1 infection.* Abstract Th.C.420, presented at the XI International Conference on AIDS, Vancouver, Canada, 7–12 July 1996.

Stimson GV, Alldritt L, Dolan K, Donoghoe M. (1988) Syringe exchange schemes for drug users in England and Scotland. *British Medical Journal* 296:1717–1719.

Susser E, Valencia E, Conover S. (1993) Prevalence of HIV infection among psychiatric patients in a New York City men's shelter. *American Journal of Public Health* April; 83: 568–570.

Swiss S, Giller JE. (1993) Rape as a crime of war. *Journal of the American Medical Association* 270:612–615.

Tabor E, Gerety RJ, Cairns J, Bayley AC. (1990) Did HIV and HTLV originate in Africa? (letter) *Journal of the American Medical Association* 264:691–692.

Tabor MBW. (1993) Judge orders release of Haitians detained in Guantanamo camp. *New York Times* 9 June 1993, p. A1.

Thomas C. (1987) *A synopsis of state AIDS-related legislation, January to July 1987.* Intergovernmental Health Policy Project. Washington, DC: George Washington University.

Thomas PA, Costigan RS. (1992) Health care or punishment? Prisoners with HIV/AIDS. *The Howard Journal of Criminal Justice* 31(4):321–336.

Tomasevski K. (1995) "Health." In: *United Nations Legal Order.* Cambridge, MA: Cambridge University Press. vol. II, pp. 859, 861, 862.

Toubia N. (1994) Female circumcision as a public health issue. *New England Journal of Medicine* 331:712–716.

Turner JC, Korpita E, Mohn LA, Hill WB. (1993) Reduction in sexual risk behaviors among college students following a comprehensive health education intervention. *College Health* 41:187–193.

United States General Accounting Office. (1993) *Needle Exchange Programs, Research Suggests Promise as an AIDS Prevention Strategy.* Report to the Chairman, Select Committee on Narcotics Abuse and Control, House of Representatives; Human Resources Division. GAO/HRD-93-60.

United States National Commission on AIDS. (1990) *Report: HIV Disease in Correctional Facilities.* Washington, DC: National Institute of Justice.

Van de Perre P, Lepage P, Homsy J, Dabis F. (1992) Mother-to-infant transmission of human immunodeficiency by breast milk: presumed innocent or presumed guilty? *Clinical Infectious Disease* 15:502–507.

Van de Perre P, Simonon A, Hitimana D-G, Dabis F, Msellati P, Mukamabano B, Butera J-B, Van Goethem C, Karita E, Lepage P. (1993) Infective and anti-infective properties of breastmilk from HIV-1–infected women. *Lancet* 341:914–918.

van den Hoek JAR, van Haastrecht HJA, Coutinho RA. (1989) Risk reduction among intravenous drug users in Amsterdam under the influence of AIDS. *American Journal of Public Health* 79:1355–1357.

Vlahov D, Munoz A, Celentano DD, Cohn S, Anthony JC, Chilcoat H, Nelson KE. (1991) HIV seroconversion and disinfection of injection equipment among intravenous drug users; Baltimore, MD. *Epidemiology* 2:444–446.

Ward JW, Holmberg SD, Allen JR, Cohn DL, Critchley SE, Kleinman SH, Lenes BA, Ravenholt O, Davis JR, Quinn MG, Jaffe HW. (1988) Transmission of human immunodeficiency virus (HIV) by blood transfusions screened as negative for HIV antibody. *New England Journal of Medicine* 318:473–478.

Watters JK. (1987) A street-based outreach model for AIDS prevention for intravenous drug users: preliminary evaluation. *Contemporary Drug Problems* 14:411–424.

Watters JK, Cheng YT, Clark GL, Lorvick J. (1991) *Syringe exchange in San Francisco: preliminary findings.* Presented at the VII International Conference on AIDS, Florence, Italy, June 1991.

Watters JK. (1994) Trends in risk behavior and HIV seroprevalence in heterosexual injection drug users in San Francisco, 1986–1992. *Journal of Acquired Immune Deficiency Syndromes* 7:1276–1281.

Wodak A, Dolan K, Imrie AA, Gold J, Wolk J, Whyte BM, Cooper DA. (1987) Antibodies to the human immunodeficiency virus in needles and syringes used by intravenous drug abusers. *Medical Journal of Australia* 147:275–276.

Wolk J, Wodak A, Gunan JJ, Macaskill P, Simpson JM. (1990) The effect of a needle and syringe exchange on a methadone maintenance unit. *British Journal of Addiction* 85:1445–1450.

Wood RW. (1990) Needle exchange programs stop AIDS! *AIDS Patient Care* 4:14–17.

Worth D. (1989) Sexual decision-making and AIDS: why condom promotion among vulnerable women is likely to fail. *Studies in Family Planning* 20:297–307.

Zeegers Paget D, Bernasconi S, Wasserfallen F, Rihs-Middel, et al. (1996) *AIDS prevention programme including needle distribution for female prisoners: the Hindelbank pilot project.* Abstract Mo.D.362, presented at the XI International Conference on AIDS, Vancouver, Canada, 7–12 July 1996.

Ziegler JB, Cooper DA, Gold J, Johnson R. (1985) Postnatal transmission of AIDS-associated retrovirus. *Lancet* 1:896–898.

Ziegler JB. (1993) Breast feeding and HIV. *Lancet* 342:1437–1438.

Appendix: Universal Declaration of Human Rights

Whereas a common understanding of these rights and freedoms is of the greatest importance for the full realization of this pledge.

Now, therefore,

The General Assembly

Proclaims this Universal Declaration of Human Rights as a common standard of achievement for all peoples and all nations, to the end that every individual and every organ of society, keeping this Declaration constantly in mind, shall strive by teaching and education to promote respect for these rights and freedoms and by progressive measures, national and international, to secure their universal and effective recognition and observance, both among the peoples of Member States themselves and among the peoples of territories under their jurisdiction.

Article 1

All human beings are born free and equal in dignity and rights. They are endowed with reason and conscience and should act towards one another in a spirit of brotherhood.

Article 2

Everyone is entitled to all the rights and freedoms set forth in this Declaration, without distinction of any kind, such as race, colour, sex, language, religion, political or other opinion, national or social origin, property, birth or other status.

Furthermore, no distinction shall be made on the basis of the political, jurisdictional or international status of the country or territory to which a person belongs, whether it be independent, trust, non-self-governing or under any other limitation of sovereignty.

Article 3

Everyone has the right to life, liberty and security of person.

Article 4

No one shall be held in slavery or servitude; slavery and the slave trade shall be prohibited in all their forms.

Article 5

No one shall be subjected to torture or to cruel, inhuman or degrading treatment or punishment.

Article 6

Everyone has the right to recognition everywhere as a person before the law.

Article 7

All are equal before the law and are entitled without any discrimination to equal protection of the law. All are entitled to equal protection against any discrimination in violation of this Declaration and against any incitement to such discrimination.

Article 8

Everyone has the right to an effective remedy by the competent national tribunals for acts violating the fundamental rights granted him by the constitution or by law.

Article 9

No one shall be subjected to arbitrary arrest, detention or exile.

Article 10

Everyone is entitled in full equality to a fair and public hearing by an independent and impartial tribunal, in the determination of his rights and obligations and of any criminal charge against him.

Article 11

1. Everyone charged with a penal offence has the right to be presumed innocent until proved guilty according to law in a public trial at which he has had all the guarantees necessary for his defence.

2. No one shall be held guilty of any penal offence on account of any act or omission which did not constitute a penal offence, under national or international law, at the time when it was committed. Nor shall a heavier penalty be imposed than the one that was applicable at the time the penal offence was committed.

Article 12

No one shall be subjected to arbitrary interference with his privacy, family, home or correspondence, nor to attacks upon his honour and reputation. Everyone has the right to the protection of the law against such interference or attacks.

Article 13

1. Everyone has the right to freedom of movement and residence within the borders of each State.
2. Everyone has the right to leave any country, including his own, and to return to his country.

Article 14

1. Everyone has the right to seek and to enjoy in other countries asylum from persecution.
2. This right may not be invoked in the case of prosecutions genuinely arising from non-political crimes or from acts contrary to the purposes and principles of the United Nations.

Article 15

1. Everyone has the right to a nationality.
2. No one shall be arbitrarily deprived of his nationality nor denied the right to change his nationality.

Article 16

1. Men and women of full age, without any limitation due to race, nationality or religion, have the right to marry and to found a family. They are entitled to equal rights as to marriage, during marriage and at its dissolution.
2. Marriage shall be entered into only with the free and full consent of the intending spouses.
3. The family is the natural and fundamental group unit of society and is entitled to protection by society and the State.

Article 17

1. Everyone has the right to own property alone as well as in association with others.
2. No one shall be arbitrarily deprived of his property.

Article 18

Everyone has the right to freedom of thought, conscience and religion; this right includes freedom to change his religion or belief, and freedom, either alone or in community with others and in public or private, to manifest his religion or belief in teaching, practice, worship and observance.

Article 19

Everyone has the right to freedom of opinion and expression; this right includes freedom to hold opinions without interference and to seek, receive and impart information and ideas through any media and regardless of frontiers.

Article 20

1. Everyone has the right to freedom of peaceful assembly and association.
2. No one may be compelled to belong to an association.

Article 21

1. Everyone has the right to take part in the government of his country, directly or through freely chosen representatives.
2. Everyone has the right of equal access to public service in his country.
3. The will of the people shall be the basis of the authority of government; this will shall be expressed in periodic and genuine elections which shall be by universal and equal suffrage and shall be held by secret vote or by equivalent free voting procedures.

Article 22

Everyone, as a member of society, has the right to social security and is entitled to realization, through national effort and international cooperation and in accordance with the organization and resources of each State, of the economic, social and cultural rights indispensable for his dignity and the free development of his personality.

Article 23

1. Everyone has the right to work, to free choice of employment, to just and favourable conditions of work and to protection against unemployment.
2. Everyone, without any discrimination, has the right to equal pay for equal work.
3. Everyone who works has the right to just and favourable remuneration ensuring for himself and his family an existence worthy of human dignity, and supplemented, if necessary, by other means of social protection.

4. Everyone has the right to form and to join trade unions for the protection of his interests.

Article 24

Everyone has the right to rest and leisure, including reasonable limitation of working hours and periodic holidays with pay.

Article 25

1. Everyone has the right to a standard of living adequate for the health and well-being of himself and of his family, including food, clothing, housing and medical care and necessary social services, and the right to security in the event of unemployment, sickness, disability, widowhood, old age or other lack of livelihood in circumstances beyond his control.

2. Motherhood and childhood are entitled to special care and assistance. All children whether born in or out of wedlock, shall enjoy the same social protection.

Article 26

1. Everyone has the right to education. Education shall be free, at least in the elementary and fundamental stages. Elementary education shall be compulsory. Technical and professional education shall be made generally available and higher education shall be equally accessible to all on the basis of merit.

2. Education shall be directed to the full development of the human personality and to the strengthening of respect for human rights and fundamental freedoms. It shall promote understanding, tolerance and friendship among all nations, racial or religious groups, and shall further the activities of the United Nations for the maintenance of peace.

3. Parents have a prior right to choose the kind of education that shall be given to their children.

Article 27

1. Everyone has the right freely to participate in the cultural life of the community, to enjoy the arts and to share in scientific advancement and its benefits.

2. Everyone has the right to the protection of the moral and material interests resulting from any scientific, literary or artistic production of which he is the author.

Article 28

Everyone is entitled to a social and international order in which the rights and freedoms set forth in this Declaration can be fully realized.

Article 29

1. Everyone has duties to the community in which alone the free and full development of his personality is possible.

2. In the exercise of his rights and freedoms, everyone shall be subject only to such limitations as are determined by law solely for the purpose of securing due recognition and respect for the rights and freedoms of others and of meeting the just requirements of morality, public order and the general welfare in a democratic society.

3. These rights and freedoms may in no case be exercised contrary to the purposes and principles of the United Nations.

Article 30

Nothing in this Declaration may be interpreted as implying for any State, group or person any right to engage in any activity or to perform any act aimed at the destruction of any of the rights and freedoms set forth herein.

Index